The periFACTS® OB/GYN Academy Presents
Fetal Heart Rate Monitoring: Pathophysiology and Practice, Third Edition

Edited by

Loralei L. Thornburg, M.D.
James R. Woods, Jr., Professor of Obstetrics and Gynecology
Associate Professor of Obstetrics and Gynecology
Director, Division of Maternal-Fetal Medicine

J. Christopher Glantz, M.D., M.P.H.
Professor of Obstetrics and Gynecology
Division of Maternal-Fetal Medicine

Kathryn Flynn, W.H.N.P.-C.
Nurse Practitioner
Department of Obstetrics and Gynecology

Candace B. Galle, R.N., B.S., C-E.FM.
Registered Nurse
Department of Obstetrics and Gynecology

and

James R. Woods, Jr., M.D.
Professor
Department of Obstetrics and Gynecology

**Department of Obstetrics and Gynecology
The University of Rochester
Rochester, New York**

Medical Editor: Leah Garnett
Indexer: Joanne Still

Contributors

Kimberlee A. Bliek, M.S., R.N., C.N.M.L., C-E.F.M.
Director, Women's Services
Multicare Deaconess Hospital
Spokane, Washington

Therese Caffery, R.N.C., M.S.N.P.
Nurse Practitioner
Department of Obstetrics and Gynecology
The University of Rochester
Rochester, New York

Jillian Dodge, M.D.
Resident
Department of Obstetrics and Gynecology
The University of Rochester
Rochester, New York

Carol Giffi, R.N.C., M.S.N.P.
Nurse Practitioner Emerita
Department of Obstetrics and Gynecology
The University of Rochester
Rochester, New York

Dzhamala Gilmandyar, M.D.
Associate Professor
Maternal-Fetal Medicine
Department of Obstetrics and Gynecology
Hackensack Meridian Medical Group
Neptune, New Jersey

Lisa Gray, M.D.
Assistant Professor
Department of Obstetrics and Gynecology
The University of Rochester
Rochester, New York

David Hackney, M.D., M.S.
Associate Professor
Division Director, Maternal-Fetal Medicine
Department of Obstetrics and Gynecology
MacDonald Women's Hospital
University Hospitals Cleveland Medical Center
Cleveland, OH

Monique Ho, M.D.
Associate Professor
Department of Obstetrics and Gynecology
The University of Rochester
Rochester, New York

Safinaz Tulin Ozcan, M.D.
Associate Professor
Maternal and Fetal Medicine
Department of Obstetrics and Gynecology
University Hospitals
Cleveland, OH

Eva K. Pressman, M.D.
Henry A. Thiede Professor and Chair
Department of Obstetrics and Gynecology
The University of Rochester
Rochester, New York

Ruth Anne Queenan, M.D., M.B.A.
Professor and Chief
Department of Obstetrics and Gynecology
Highland Hospital
Rochester, NY

Neil Seligman, M.D.
Assistant Professor
Department of Obstetrics and Gynecology
The University of Rochester
Rochester, NY

Shirley Warren, R.N.C., M.S.N.P.-B.C.
Clinical Nurse Specialist Emerita
Department of Obstetrics and Gynecology
The University of Rochester
Rochester, New York

Paula Zozzaro-Smith, D.O.
Maternal-Fetal Medicine
Department of Obstetrics and Gynecology
Baylor, Scott, and White Health
Waco, Texas

Preface

We are pleased to introduce the third edition of our periFACTS® OB/GYN Academy textbook, *Fetal Heart Rate Monitoring: Pathophysiology and Practice*. This textbook has been completely revised to update the terminology, and to include the most up-to-date information on maternal and fetal physiology and its use in interpretation of fetal assessment.

The initial chapters in this textbook focus on physiologic adaptations of pregnancy and the basic physiology of oxygen delivery to the fetus. In subsequent chapters, different aspects of fetal assessment in various clinical scenarios are reviewed. This textbook has been expanded to fully discuss fetal monitoring and interpretation.

The clinical case studies have been replaced and include new fetal heart rate tracings and questions. Many of the fetal heart rate tracings offer examples of basic fetal heart rate monitoring interpretation; others have been selected specifically for the advanced learner seeking a higher level of interpretation in more complicated fetal assessment.

Fetal Heart Rate Monitoring: Pathophysiology and Practice is the core reference textbook for the periFACTS® OB/GYN Academy Obstetrics and Fetal Monitoring course.

For more information regarding all the offerings of the periFACTS® OB/GYN Academy and our other textbooks, online learning opportunities, videos, and women's health content, visit our web site at www.perifacts.urmc.edu. Input always is welcome from those who utilize this textbook, and we hope that it serves as a worthy resource within your obstetric practice.

Table of Contents

Chapter 4
Fetal Oxygen and Acid-Base Metabolism

Chapter 5
Amniotic Fluid Physiology

Chapter 6
Assessment of Uterine Activity

Chapter 7
Fetal Heart Rate Monitoring: Technology, Baseline, and Variability

Chapter 8
Accelerations and Decelerations

Chapter 9
Antepartum Fetal Assessment

Chapter 10
Fetal Heart Rate Monitoring Interpretation

Chapter 11
Fetal Assessment by Doppler Velocimetry

Chapter 12
Fetal Monitoring in the Complex Patient

Chapter 13
Patient Safety and Team Communication:
Developing a Culture of Safety and Teamwork

Chapter 14
Putting It All Together:
Basic Fetal Heart Rate Monitor Interpretation Case Studies

Chapter 15
Putting It All Together:
Advanced Fetal Heart Rate Monitor Interpretation Case Studies

Chapter 1

Maternal Pregnancy Physiology and Initiation of Parturition

- ◆ Introduction
- ◆ Reproductive System
- ◆ Cardiovascular System
- ◆ Hematologic Changes
- ◆ Respiratory Changes
- ◆ Renal Function
- ◆ Labor and Myometrial Function
- ◆ Conclusion
- ◆ Related Readings
- ◆ Review

INTRODUCTION

Imagine your next patient is a 35-year-old woman with multiple complaints, including nausea and vomiting, heartburn, constipation, weight gain, backache, amenorrhea, and urinary frequency. She also complains of fatigue, palpitations, shortness of breath, leg swelling, occasional syncope, and areas of darkened skin. Vital signs include hypotension with a blood pressure of 100/50 mmHg. She has a mild systolic ejection murmur along the left sternal border.

Laboratory evaluation reveals mild anemia and leukocytosis. Her fibrinogen is high and her electrolytes are consistent with mild acidosis. Her alkaline phosphatase is 150 IU/L and she has low serum albumin and glucosuria. Arterial blood gas values reveal a compensated pH of 7.40, PCO_2 of 30 mmHg, and PO_2 of 104 mmHg.

A chest x-ray shows an elevated diaphragm and borderline cardiomegaly. An electrocardiogram reveals left axis deviation, and an echocardiogram reveals increased cardiac output. Pulmonary function tests show increased tidal volume but decreased residual capacity. A renal sonogram shows mild bilateral hydronephrosis, which is worse on the right.

Chances are this patient would be considered ill by most providers, but for those who provide routine obstetric care, these are the normal physiologic changes of pregnancy. Most of the laboratory values presented above would be considered abnormal in a nonpregnant woman, but all can be explained by the physiologic adaptations of the body to pregnancy. A woman's body actually adapts itself to pregnancy with the imperative of facilitating growth and development of a new human being. The changes visible externally and the myriad of physiologic adjustments taking place internally serve to create this optimal environment for the fetus.

REPRODUCTIVE SYSTEM

The uterus undergoes estrogen-induced hypertrophy unprecedented in any other organ system, increasing its weight from 70 grams to 1,100 grams, expanding capacity 500- to 1,000-fold. The uterus is dextrorotated slightly, partly because the left-sided rectosigmoid colon compresses the uterus asymmetrically with the right receiving more pressure than the left. The uterus is functionally denervated at term but still has adrenergic receptors and can respond to hematogenous catecholamines.

The cervix softens, appears cyanotic, and undergoes glandular proliferation during pregnancy. The transformation zone everts, and the exposed glandular tissue may bleed more easily. Within the ovary, the site of ovulation, the corpus luteum produces progesterone to maintain the developing pregnancy until approximately eight to ten weeks' post-conception, after which time the placenta is able to completely take over this function and the corpus luteum no longer is necessary.

CARDIOVASCULAR SYSTEM

Fetal growth and development depend on adequate delivery of oxygen and nutrients, and on satisfactory excretion of waste. Oxygen and nutrients must be supplied through the maternal circulation, which in turn must carry away waste products. In the nonpregnant state, food intake, respiration, hemoglobin oxygen-carrying capacity, and cardiac output match the individual's needs. In pregnancy, these needs increase because of the additional fetal requirements, and, therefore, the cardiovascular system adapts accordingly.

Cardiac output equals heart rate times stroke volume (CO = HR x SV). Stroke volume is the amount of blood ejected by the heart during each ventricular contraction. Baseline heart rate increases by 10 to 15 beats per minute (bpm) during pregnancy, and improved cardiac contractility augments stroke volume. Heart size increases by approximately 12%. The combined effect is an eventual 30% to 50% increase in cardiac output beginning in the first trimester, circulating blood more effectively (see Figure 1.1). This increased flow through the heart causes turbulence and produces the benign systolic murmurs commonly heard during pregnancy. Cardiac output also may increase during labor partly because, with every uterine contraction, 300 to 500 mL of uterine blood is forced into the maternal venous circulation, further increasing stroke volume. This increased cardiac output can be seen on echocardiography.

Figure 1.1: Changes in heart rate, stroke volume, and cardiac output with increasing gestational age. The left axis refers to heart rate (dark line) and stroke volume (thin line), and the right axis refers to the percent change in cardiac output (dotted line). Note the changes occur early in pregnancy.

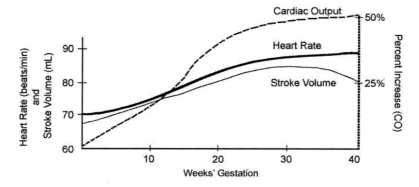

The expansion of intravascular volume during pregnancy also results in major changes in cardiac output. Cardiac output (CO) is the product of heart rate (HR) and stroke volume (SV): CO = HR x SV. Maternal heart rate increases by approximately 20% by term (15 to 20 bpm). At 20 to 24 weeks' gestation, stroke volume is increased by 25% and by 30 weeks is increased by 50%. Cardiac output is influenced by many other variables and clinical situations (Table 1.1). Labor, multiple gestation, infections, and various drug therapies all increase cardiac output from the baseline of 6 to 7 L/min.

Any amount of blood the heart pumps out must first be taken in. This flow is the *venous return* through the vena cava into the right atrium. When the inferior vena cava is compressed by the enlarged gravid uterus in the supine woman, venous flow decreases, less blood returns to the heart, cardiac output falls, and the woman becomes hypotensive. This represents *supine hypotension,* seen when a pregnant woman in the latter half of pregnancy lies flat on her back. The drop in blood pressure may lead to a vasovagal response in the mother (parasympathetic slowing of the heart rate, accompanied by nausea and fainting) and inadequate uteroplacental perfusion. It is relieved easily by turning the woman to her side to move the uterus off the vena cava, restoring flow. Uterine compression of pelvic veins also slows venous return from the extremities. Coupled with increased plasma volume and low

Table 1.1: Positional Effects on Cardiac Output

Position	Cardiac Output (L/min)
Knee chest	6.9
Right side	6.8
Left side	6.6
Sitting	6.2
Supine	6.0
Standing	5.4

Adapted from "Position change and central hemodynamic profile during normal third-trimester pregnancy and postpartum," American Journal of Obstetrics and Gynecology (1991).

plasma oncotic pressure from decreased serum albumin concentrations, increased venous pressure forces fluid across vessel walls into peripheral tissues, causing dependent edema.

Blood pressure equals *blood flow* times *resistance* (BP = F x R). Total flow is the same as cardiac output, while resistance is the friction the blood encounters in the vessels. Systemic vascular resistance falls due to the low resistance of the placenta and the action of progesterone, prostaglandins, and estrogen-induced nitric oxide on the vessels and this decrease in resistance proportionally is greater than the increase in flow. Diastolic

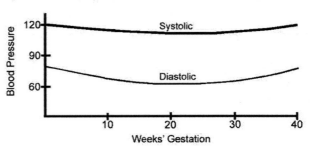

Figure 1.2: Changes in Blood Pressure with Gestational Age

blood pressure falls 10 to 15 mmHg by mid-pregnancy (although it tends to rise back up to baseline by term: see Figure 1.2). **This allows greater flow at lower pressure, minimizing cardiac work.**

Because the enlarging uterus pushes upward on the abdominal contents, which subsequently push upward on the diaphragm, chest x-ray often shows elevation of the diaphragm and deviation of the heart towards the left. This deviation of the heart may give the impression of cardiomegaly on a chest x-ray and also results in deviation of the electrical axis to the left during electrocardiography.

HEMATOLOGIC CHANGES

Concurrent with these changes in flow, the blood itself undergoes transformation that is evident by the end of the first trimester. Hemoglobin in red blood cells (RBC) transports oxygen. Although erythropoietin generally increases in response to low oxygen, levels increase despite an increase in PO_2. This increase stimulates the bone marrow to produce 20% to 30% more RBCs than in the nonpregnant state and serves to improve the capacity of blood to convey oxygen to the fetus.

Figure 1.3: Increase in Blood Volume and RBC Mass as Pregnancy Progresses. Although RBC mass increases, it is diluted by an even greater increase in blood volume so that the pregnant woman's hematocrit falls.

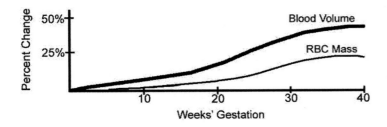

Blood has a certain "thickness" termed viscosity, which provides some of the friction to flow. The thicker the fluid, the more friction to flow (think of honey on a spoon); the more dilute the fluid, the less friction. The higher the blood viscosity, the slower the flow and the greater the tendency to sludge in the vessels, predisposing to thrombosis. Red blood cells increase blood viscosity; to counteract this effect, the body increases the amount of fluid or plasma in the blood by approximately 50% to dilute the RBCs and decrease friction.

The 50% increase in plasma volume outweighs the 20 to 30% increase in RBCs, so that the patient appears "anemic" because of the dilutional effect, even though she has more RBCs than she had before pregnancy (Figure 1.3). This increase in fluid is due partially to vasodilation and partially to sodium retention mediated by increases in renin-aldosterone, beginning in the first trimester. The end results are greater oxygen-carrying capacity due to increased hemoglobin and cardiac output, and decreased friction (further facilitating increased flow) due to dilution of the blood by increased plasma volume. Other benefits of volume expansion and increased RBC mass are dissipation of maternal-fetal heat, increased renal filtration, and a reserve for the inevitable loss of blood that occurs at delivery.

Table 1.2: Hematologic Laboratory Assessment during Pregnancy

Test	Nonpregnant	Pregnant
Hematocrit	37% to 47%	33% to 44%
Hemoglobin	12 to 16 g/dL	11 to 14 g/dL
WBC count	4.5 to 11 x10^3/mm^3	6 to 16 x10^3/ mm^3
Platelet count	130 to 400 x10^3/ mm^3	Slight decrease
Fibrinogen	200 to 450 mg/dL	400 to 650 mg/dL
Prothrombin time (PT)	12 to 14 sec	Unchanged
Partial thromboplastin time (PTT)	24 to 36 sec	Unchanged

Adapted from Burrow and Duffy, 1999.

Hematocrits as low as approximately 33% are considered normal in pregnancy (Table 1.2); hematocrits below 33% may be an accentuated "physiologic" anemia (nonpathologic), may be due to iron-deficiency anemia common in many women, or occasionally may represent hemoglobinopathies or unusual pathologic conditions. A simple way of differentiating the first two entities is by assessing serum ferritin concentration. Ferritin is a molecule that binds iron, and ferritin's concentration is proportional roughly to body iron stores. Normal ferritin is inconsistent with iron deficiency anemia, except when an inflammatory condition such as lupus nephritis is present (inflammation elevates ferritin concentrations regardless of iron stores). Hemoglobinopathies can be ruled out by hemoglobin electrophoresis, and folate or B_{12} deficiency anemia can be assessed by serum concentrations of the vitamins. The white blood cell (WBC) count rises slightly in pregnancy, up to as high as 16,000/mm^3. Most of these additional WBCs are granulocytes, also known as polymorphonuclear leukocytes (PMNs) responsible for humoral immunity.

RESPIRATORY CHANGES

Oxygen is essential for metabolism and energy production. Because of increased gestational metabolic requirements and the presence of the fetus, oxygen consumption increases 15 to 20% during pregnancy. To accommodate such an increase, progesterone acts on the respiratory centers within the central nervous system to increase minute ventilation (the amount of air breathed in and out in one minute) by 30% to 40%, primarily by increasing tidal volume (the volume of a normal breath) rather than by accelerating the respiratory rate. This maximizes oxygen transport into the blood and hastens diffusion of carbon dioxide (CO_2) out of the blood. Coupled with the increase in hemoglobin and its oxygen-binding capacity, the result is higher PO_2 and lower PCO_2 in maternal blood. This means that the gradient between maternal and fetal blood favors transfer of O_2 to the fetus, and transfer of CO_2 out of the fetus into the maternal circulation. Despite this physiologic hyperventilation, renal bicarbonate excretion prevents maternal pH from rising.

Although ventilation increases in pregnancy, many pregnant women complain of dyspnea. Estrogen causes edema and erythema of the nasal mucosa, predisposing to congestion and nosebleeds. The enlarging uterus pushes up on the diaphragm, impinging on the reserve volume of the lungs. Although tidal volume is increased, there is less reserve volume if the woman tries to take a deep breath. High oxygen consumption and lower reserve volumes during pregnancy also make pregnant women susceptible to rapid development of hypoxemia if there is compromise of the airway.

RENAL FUNCTION

Fetal kidneys produce urine, which is excreted into the amniotic fluid. If this were the only way the fetus could clear waste materials, the amniotic fluid soon would be filled with waste. However, unlike in the adult, most wastes do not pass into the amniotic fluid but instead cross the placenta into maternal blood and are excreted by the maternal kidneys.

The ability of the maternal renal glomeruli to filter waste products out of the blood depends on blood flow through the kidney. Because maternal kidneys are presented with greater amounts of waste products to clear, it is beneficial that increased cardiac output means that more blood flows through the kidneys per unit of time during pregnancy. This *renal plasma flow* increases up to 75% above nonpregnant levels. Higher renal plasma flow increases the *glomerular filtration rate (GFR)* by approximately 50%, increasing the efficiency by which the kidneys filter the blood. This does not mean that more urine actually is produced. Renal tubular fluid reabsorption also is increased during pregnancy to prevent urinary loss of necessary fluids, proteins, and metabolites. Aldosterone concentrations increase two- to three-fold during pregnancy and help facilitate this reabsorption. Additional sodium reabsorption increases due to increased aldosterone and deoxycorticosterone. This results in a drop in plasma osmolality by approximately 10 mOsm. Protein excretion is unchanged during normal pregnancy.

Increased GFR allows creatinine and blood urea nitrogen (BUN)—nitrogenous wastes that are produced in greater amounts during pregnancy because of combined maternal-fetal metabolism—to be filtered in greater quantities than during the nonpregnant state. Increased filtration more than compensates for increased waste production; therefore, serum creatinine and BUN concentrations during pregnancy are approximately half of what they would be during the nonpregnant state (Table 1.3). Creatinine clearance (a measure of the ability of the kidney to filter creatinine) rises from 100 mL/min to greater than 150 mL/min. This over-compensation creates a gradient for waste across the maternal-fetal unit. Just as the drop in maternal PCO_2 from 40 mmHg to approximately 30 mmHg during pregnancy creates a CO_2 gradient across the fetal-maternal unit gradient and drives CO_2 exchange from fetal to maternal blood, lowering maternal serum creatinine concentration promotes transfer of creatinine waste from fetal to maternal blood.

Table 1.3: Renal Laboratory Assessment during Pregnancy

Test	Nonpregnant	Pregnant
Creatinine	<1.5 mg/dL	<0.8 mg/dL
BUN	10 to 20 mg/dL	5 to 12 mg/dL
Sodium	136 to 145 mEq/L	130 to 140 mEq/L
Potassium	3.5 to 5.0 mEq/L	3.3 to 4.1 mEq/L
CO_2 content	21 to 30 mEq/L	18 to 25 mEq/L
Calcium	9.0 to 10.5 mg/dL	8.1 to 9.5 mg/dL
Glucose (fasting)	75 to 115 mg/dL	60 to 105 mg/dL
Uric acid	1.5 to 6.0 mg/dL	1.2 to 4.5 mg/dL

Adapted from Burrow and Duffy, 1999.

Glucose normally is filtered in the proximal tubule of the glomeruli, and most of the filtered glucose is reabsorbed in the distal tubule. Increased volume of filtrate presented to the tubules during pregnancy may exceed the glucose-reabsorbing capacity, leading to glucosuria. Glucosuria would be of concern in the nonpregnant state but is less of a concern during pregnancy. Although persistent glucosuria should lead to testing of maternal carbohydrate tolerance to rule out diabetes, the majority of such cases are normal.

A combination of progesterone mediated ureteral smooth-muscle relaxation and compression of the ureters by the enlarging uterus may cause mild obstructive hydronephrosis (dilation of the renal pelvis and calyces) during pregnancy. Because of the dextrorotation of the uterus (dextro=right), the right ureter tends to be compressed more than the left. As long as the hydronephrosis is mild, this is considered within normal limits for pregnancy. Moderate-to-severe hydronephrosis should lead to consideration of pathologic obstructions such as renal stones, congenital abnormalities, and may warrant further intervention.

LABOR AND MYOMETRIAL FUNCTION

Labor fundamentally consists of regular uterine contractions of sufficient strength at regular intervals which lead to cervical dilation and effacement and eventual amniotic membrane rupture and expulsion of the fetus. How this occurs, the initiation and timing, is complex.

In addition to the uterus' serosal exterior and endometrial lining, it primarily consists of muscle cells called myometrium. Like all muscles in the human body, uterine contractions are fundamentally dependent upon the interactions between the "motor protein" myocin and the actin filaments. Myocin is "activated" when it is phosphoralated (the attachment of a phosphate group) by a protein known as "MLCK" or "myosin light chain kinase" (a "kinase" is a protein which attaches a phosphate group to other proteins). MLCK, in turn, is activated or deactivated through a variety of mechanisms, and it primarily is through this process that uterine contractile activity is controlled. For example, increased intracellular calcium concentrations stimulate MLCK, which is why calcium-channel blockers may inhibit preterm labor. The primary process of myometrial contraction activation is through increased intracellular calcium secondary to stimulation by prostaglandins. Prostaglandins themselves can be generated through a variety of processes. They naturally are present in seminal fluid (the name "prostaglandin" is derived from the word "prostate gland"), which is why pregnant women will often contract after sexual intercourse. Prostaglandin production by the uterus and fetal membranes increase at term as one of the primary stimulators of term labor, though prior to term it also can be generated by a variety of pathologic processes such as bleeding or infection.

In addition to the activation of myocin within the individual muscle fibers, the process of labor also requires that the different muscle cells within the uterus coordinate themselves in order to produce uterine-wide contractions that occur in a regular and synchronized manner. This process requires the formation of collections of proteins known as "gap junction proteins" whose purpose is to form tiny aqueous channels between adjacent myometrial cells through which electrolytes and electrical changes can flow. The primary gap junction protein in the uterus is called "Connexin-43," the expression of which is increased when myometrial cells experience mechanical stretch. Normally, this occurs near term in preparation for labor; however, in cases of twins and other multifetal gestations, excessive mechanical stretch in early pregnancy can stimulate the premature expression of Connexin-43.

CONCLUSION

Many physiologic changes occur during pregnancy, and many of these manifest themselves in different ranges-of-normal for laboratory results—results that would be considered abnormal in the nonpregnant state. It is not uncommon for care providers who are inexperienced in caring for obstetric patients to become very concerned when laboratory values are outside the normal (nonpregnant) range. This can lead to unwarranted further testing, consultation, treatment, and patient and provider anxiety. It is important to understand the physiology changes during pregnancy, and how these changes influence interpretation of laboratory test results. It also is important to understand that the "normal" ranges printed alongside most laboratory results represent what would be normal for nonpregnant individuals, not what would be normal for pregnancy.

RELATED READINGS

1. Burrow GN and Duffy TP (1999). <u>Medical Complications during Pregnancy</u> (Ed. 5), Philadelphia, PA: W.B. Saunders Company.

2. Cheek TG and Gutsche BB (2002). Maternal physiologic alterations during pregnancy. IN: SC Hughes, G Levinson, MA and Rosen (Eds.), <u>Anesthesia for Obstetrics</u> (Ed. 4), Baltimore, MD: Williams and Wilkins, pp. 3-18.

3. Cunningham FG, Leveno KJ, Bloom SL, Hauth JC, Gilstrap LC, and Wenstrom KD (2005). Maternal physiology (Chapter 5). IN: <u>Williams Obstetrics</u> (Ed. 22), Norwalk, CT: McGraw Hill Companies, Inc., pp. 121-150.

4. Wallach J (2000). <u>Interpretation of Diagnostic Tests</u> (Ed. 7), Philadelphia, PA: Lippincott Williams and Wilkins.

Chapter 1 Review
Maternal Pregnancy Physiology and Initiation of Parturition

1. During pregnancy, changes to the maternal cardiovascular system include:

    A. decreased heart rate.
    B. improved cardiac contractility.
    C. increased size of the heart.
    D. increased cardiac output of 30% to 50%.
    E. all of the above.
    F. A and B only.
    G. B, C, and D only.

2. During normal pregnancy, mid-trimester diastolic blood pressure:

    A. increases.
    B. decreases.
    C. remains the same.

3. The hematologic value that remains unchanged during a normal pregnancy is:

    A. hematocrit.
    B. hemoglobin.
    C. white blood cell count.
    D. platelet count.
    E. fibrinogen.
    F. prothrombin time/partial thromboplastin time (International Normalized Ratio).

4. True or False. The majority of glucosuria in pregnancy is normal.

    A. True
    B. False

5. One of the primary stimulators of term labor is:

    A. estrogen.
    B. progesterone.
    C. prostaglandin.
    D. human chorionic gonadotropin.

Chapter 1 Review Answers
Maternal Pregnancy Physiology
and Initiation of Parturition

1. **The correct answer is G.** The maternal heart rate is increased by 10 to 15 bpm. The increased heart rate coupled with improved cardiac contractility result in an eventual 30% to 50% increase in cardiac output.

2. **The correct answer is B.** Diastolic blood pressure falls 10 to 15 mmHg by mid-pregnancy due to the decrease in systemic vascular resistance.

3. **The correct answer is F.**

4. **The correct answer is A.** The increase in volume of filtrate presented to the renal tubules during pregnancy may exceed their glucose absorbing capacity, resulting in glucosuria.

5. **The correct answer is C.** Prostaglandins stimulate myometrial contractions through increased intracellular calcium.

Chapter 2

Fluid Dynamics in Pregnancy

INTRODUCTION

Maintaining proper tissue water and circulatory volume is the goal of body fluid homeostasis. During pregnancy, significant expansion of intravascular volume is required to maintain health of both the mother and the fetus. With insufficient expansion, outcomes suffer. If intravascular fluid is lost (bleeding or dehydration), adequate replacement is required to maintain tissue oxygenation. If done incorrectly, the consequences can be devastating and possibly lethal to the fetus or mother. This chapter briefly reviews fluid and electrolyte dynamics, and discusses basic fluid and electrolyte management during pregnancy. Understanding these principles improves management decisions, both for healthy pregnant women as well as those who are critically ill.

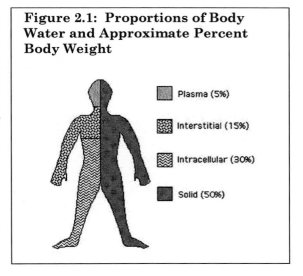

Figure 2.1: Proportions of Body Water and Approximate Percent Body Weight

- Plasma (5%)
- Interstitial (15%)
- Intracellular (30%)
- Solid (50%)

DISTRIBUTION OF FLUIDS

Water is the most common component of the human body, accounting for 50% of body weight. Total body water (TBW) is distributed into two major compartments: intracellular fluid and extracellular fluid. Intracellular fluid accounts for approximately two thirds of TBW and extracellular fluid for the remaining one third (Figure 2.1). Extracellular fluid can be further divided into two compartments: intravascular fluid and extravascular fluid, the latter known as interstitial fluid/space. There is constant flux between the compartments and wide variations between individuals, so these proportions are estimates.

KEYWORDS

Colloid Osmotic Pressure:	Osmotic pressure exerted by proteins
Extracellular:	Outside the cells
Extravascular:	Outside the blood vessels
Interstitial:	Between the cells
Intracellular:	Inside the cells
Intravascular:	Inside the blood vessels
Hydrostatic Pressure:	Pressure of fluid (e.g., blood pressure)
Hypertonic Fluids:	Fluids having a higher concentration of solutes than serum
Hypotonic Fluids:	Fluids having a lower concentration of solutes than serum
Osmolarity:	Amount of a solute in a liter of solution
Osmolality:	Amount of solute in a liter of solvent (similar, but not identical to, osmolarity)
Osmosis:	Process by which water (versus solute) diffuses through a membrane from a lower to a higher solute concentration
Osmotic Pressure:	The driving force for movement of solvent and solutes from different concentrations
Solutes:	Electrolytes and larger molecular substances, such as proteins.
Solvent:	In biologic systems, water.

Flow of water from compartment to compartment occurs through semipermeable membranes and is determined by osmotic and hydrostatic pressures. Osmosis is the process by which water diffuses through a membrane. This requires a difference across the membrane in the concentration of a molecule (solute) that cannot traverse the membrane, creating a concentration gradient. Osmotically active particles in solution govern osmotic pressure, and the gradient pulls water into the compartment with the higher concentration of solute in an effort to equalize concentrations.

MEASUREMENT OF FLUIDS, ELECTROLYTES, AND CONCENTRATIONS

A mole is a unit of measurement equaling 6×10^{23} molecules, and one millimole (mmol) is 1/1,000 of a mole. Body fluids contain relatively small amounts of solute. These can be measured in milliequivalents (mEq) based on their electrical charge, or as mmols based on the number of molecules. Osmolarity is the number of moles of solute particles dissolved per unit fluid volume (e.g., liter). Osmolality is the number of moles of particles dissolved in a mass of fluid (e.g., in 1,000 grams of water). If a liter container contains 50 gm of salt and one adds enough water to make an even liter, the amount of water added to the container will be slightly less than 1,000 mL, and the resulting salt concentration will be expressed as osmolarity. If one adds exactly 1 liter of water to a second container also containing 50 gm of salt, the total volume now will be just over 1,000 mL due to the combined volume of salt and water. This would be expressed as osmolality.

"Equivalents" refer to the number of moles of ions multiplied by the absolute value of the ion's charge. When the charge equals 1 (e.g., Na^{+1} or Cl^{-1}), the number of equivalents equals the number of moles of molecules. When the charge equals 2 (e.g., Ca^{+2} or SO_4^{-2}), the number of equivalents equals twice the number of moles (Eq = mols x absolute value of charge). Thus 1 mole of NaCl contains 1 Eq of sodium, while 1 mole of $CaSO_4$ contains 0.5 Eq of calcium. This somewhat confusing concept has to do with the balance of electrical charges during combination reactions.

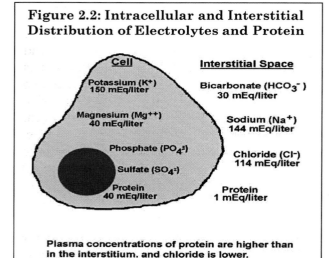

Figure 2.2: Intracellular and Interstitial Distribution of Electrolytes and Protein

Cell

Potassium (K⁺)
150 mEq/liter

Magnesium (Mg⁺⁺)
40 mEq/liter

Phosphate (PO₄⁻)

Sulfate (SO₄⁻)

Protein
40 mEq/liter

Interstitial Space

Bicarbonate (HCO₃⁻)
30 mEq/liter

Sodium (Na⁺)
144 mEq/liter

Chloride (Cl⁻)
114 mEq/liter

Protein
1 mEq/liter

Plasma concentrations of protein are higher than in the interstitium. and chloride is lower.

Electrolytes and larger molecular substances, such as proteins, are the major solutes in body fluids (Figure 2.2). Sodium (Na^+) is the primary solute responsible for osmotic "pull" in extracellular fluid. Maintaining its concentration in the intravascular space is critical in maintaining adequate intravascular volume. Potassium (K^+) and phosphates are the major intracellular solutes. At the capillary level, protein concentrations also are critical in fluid movements.

OSMOSIS

In clinical practice, there are two main types of osmotic pressure gradients: those caused by crystalloids (solutions containing salt) and those caused by colloids (solutions containing proteins). Colloid osmotic pressure (COP) is the specific type of osmotic pressure exerted by proteins. When all body fluids have equivalent solute concentration, there is no "pulling" effect on water, and these fluids, therefore, are isotonic. Hypertonic fluids have higher concentrations of solutes. Hypotonic fluids have lower concentration of solutes. Decisions regarding administration of intravenous fluids require consideration of the fluid's osmolarity (Table 2.1).

Movement of water between the intravascular space and the interstitial space occurs primarily at the level of the capillary beds. In a typical healthy individual, capillary membranes are permeable to water and many electrolytes, thus these are freely mobile. Capillary membranes are relatively

Table 2.1: Intravenous Fluid Solution Osmolarity

Solution	Osmolarity mOsm/L	Relationship to Intravascular Fluid
0.9% saline	308	Isotonic
0.45% saline	154	Hypotonic
Ringer's lactate	273	Isotonic

impermeable to proteins, though, so proteins create a gradient between the higher-protein blood and lower-protein interstitium, resulting in osmotic disequilibrium. Concurrently, hydrostatic pressure "pushes" water from blood vessels towards lower-pressure interstitial spaces, thus movement of water across the capillary membrane depends on a balance between COP and hydrostatic pressure. On the arteriolar side of the capillary bed, higher capillary blood pressure pushes water out of the vessel, while higher plasma COP pulls water inward.

Usually, oncotic pressure does not change as blood flows through a capillary, and hydrostatic pressure in the interstitial space is relatively constant. There is, however, a lessening of intra-capillary hydrostatic pressure as blood flows from arterioles to venules. Pressure decreases as fluid moves away from the left ventricle, resulting in water moving from the interstitium into the intravascular compartment. Fluid remaining in the interstitium is then removed by lymphatic drainage and returned to the circulation.

HEMODYNAMIC CHANGES IN PREGNANCY

Total body fluid increases to between 6.5 L and 8.5 L during pregnancy, with plasma volume increasing by 50% in the first trimester and plateauing by 33 to 34 weeks' gestation. Plasma volume increases even more in multiple gestations. Much of the increase in plasma volume is secondary to vasodilation. Vasodilation is caused mainly by an increase in the hormones progesterone, prostacyclin, and nitric oxide, and a decreased sensitivity to angiotensin. Vasodilation results in increased plasma renin activity and decreased atrial natriuretic protein. The net result is renal retention of sodium by enhanced tubular reabsorption. Despite this, plasma Na^+ concentration actually decreases by 3 to 5 mEq/dL, because the central hypothalamic osmotic threshold is reset and there is increased fluid retention. Osmolality decreases by 8 to 10 mOsm/L starting as early as eight weeks' gestation. Thus, attempts to "correct" plasma Na^+ to nonpregnant norms are inappropriate.

Colloid osmotic pressure also is decreased during pregnancy (Table 2.2). The intravascular proteins, albumin, globulin, and fibrinogen are diluted by the increased water within the intravascular space. This dilution results in greater potential for fluid movement into the interstitial space, predisposing pregnant patients to edema, such as that commonly encountered in the lower extremities. Pulmonary edema occurs when water flows into the pulmonary interstitial space. Bleeding and preeclampsia both lower colloid oncotic pressure further by depleting intravascular proteins. During intravenous fluid infusion, COP is further decreased by approximately 10% per liter of isotonic crystalloid solution administered.

Table 2.2: Estimates of Colloid Osmotic Pressure

	COP mmHg
Nonpregnant	25.4 ± 2.3
Antepartum	22.4 ± 0.5
Postpartum	15.4 ± 2.1
Antepartum + Preeclampsia	17.9 ± 0.7
Postpartum + Preeclampsia	13.7 ± 0.5

Adapted from "Critical Care Obstetrics" (2004, p 348) and "Studies of colloid osmotic pressure in pregnancy-induced hypertension," American Journal of Obstetrics and Gynecology (1979).

ELECTROLYTES

Salts are formed by combinations of molecules with positive or negative charges (*ions*) that electrically balance. For example, sodium has one positive charge and chloride has one negative charge, so sodium chloride electrically is neutral. Salt concentrations commonly are expressed as *equivalents*, the measure of the number of electrical charges present. Because one equivalent is a very large number of atoms, most salt concentrations are expressed as milliequivalents (*mEq*, or 1/1,000 of an equivalent, albeit still a very large number of actual molecules).

Specific gravity is a measure of the weight of solute in water, rather than actual concentration. Higher specific gravity means greater weight of solute in the solution. Because specific gravity is related to particle weight as well as number of particles, light molecules (e.g., urea) will have lower specific gravities than the same concentration of heavier molecules (e.g., glucose). Thus, unless one knows the exact composition of the solution (unlikely in the case of urine), specific gravity may under- or over-estimate true osmolality. However, as an approximation, the higher the specific gravity, the more concentrated the urine usually is.

Tonicity refers to the amount of particles dissolved in solution relative to particles dissolved within cells or serum. *Isotonic* solutions have the same osmolality as serum. *Hypotonic* solutions are more dilute than serum, and *hyper*tonic solutions are more concentrated. Pure water is maximally hypotonic; cells exposed to pure water absorb it, swell, and burst (osmotic shock). In contrast, concentrated saline is very hypertonic and draws water out of cells, causing them to dehydrate and shrivel.

Sodium

Most adults ingest between 3 to 5 gm (50 to 90 mEq) of sodium per day through diet. Sodium is lost through urine, sweat, and stool, with the kidneys tightly regulating total body concentrations to maintain extracellular fluid balance. Pregnant women retain sodium, but then dilute it with even greater degrees of water retention. Elevated serum sodium concentrations (hypernatremia, [Na] greater than 145 mEq/L) may be due to losses of dilute fluid from profuse sweating or diarrhea, decreased water intake, osmotic diuresis from glucose or mannitol (solutes excreted through the urine, pulling water along with them and leaving salts behind), hyperaldosteronism (excess adrenal mineralocorticoids that cause sodium retention), or from diabetes insipidus due to lack of pituitary antidiuretic hormone (ADH, which causes the kidney to retain water). Diabetes insipidus can follow episodes of profound hypotension after obstetric hemorrhage, resulting in infarction of the pituitary gland (Sheehan's syndrome). Overly aggressive administration of intravenous hypertonic saline is another cause of hypernatremia.

Low serum sodium concentrations (hyponatremia, [Na] less than 135 mEq/L when not pregnant, or less than 125 to 130 mEq/L when pregnant) are more common than hypernatremia, and may be due to gastrointestinal sodium losses (vomiting or diarrhea), sodium loss from diuretics, hydration with hypotonic solutions, heart/liver/renal/adrenal failure, severe hypothyroidism, excessive water retention from inappropriate secretion of ADH, or with ingestion of large quantities of water (polydipsia). Excessive water retention with resulting hyponatremia may occur after prolonged use of high-dose oxytocin due to its ADH-like pharmacologic effects. Hyperglycemia and normal-osmolal hyperlipidemia or hyperproteinemia can lower measured sodium concentration, either because glucose draws water into the plasma and dilutes sodium (by 2.4 mEq/L per 100 mg/dL rise in glucose) or because lipids or proteins occupy a greater volume of plasma, resulting in a lower volume of water in which to dissolve sodium.

For most patients, mild degrees of sodium imbalance usually are well tolerated, and acute changes in sodium are more likely to be symptomatic than are chronic changes. Severely high or low serum sodium concentrations are dangerous and can cause seizures, stupor, or coma due to osmotic movement of water out of or into brain cells, resulting in neuronal dehydration or swelling. Therapy for sodium imbalance involves treating the underlying disorder, followed by slow infusion of hypotonic fluid (with or without sodium-excreting diuretics) in the case of hypernatremia, and fluid restriction or pharmacologic diuresis while slowly administering isotonic saline in cases of hyponatremia. Sodium levels should be brought back to normal gradually. Rapid restoration of normal values can lead to neurologic injury, either from cerebral edema in the case of overly aggressive correction of hypernatremia, or demyelination from osmotic shrinkage of neurons in the case of hyponatremia. In general, it is best to aim for corrections in serum sodium concentration of 10 mEq/L per day.

Potassium

Potassium intake ranges from 50 to 100 mEq per day, and 98% of body potassium is inside cells. Potassium concentrations are regulated tightly by the kidneys; the normal range of serum potassium in the body is 3.5 to 5.0 mEq/L. Because potassium is present in small amounts only in the extracellular space, this ion's primary role is in intracellular processes rather than osmotic regulation. Elevated serum potassium (hyperkalemia) occurs during acidosis (acidic protons enter cells in exchange for potassium ions which leave the cells), renal failure/ACE inhibitors/potassium-sparing diuretics (potassium not excreted by the kidney), hypoaldosteronism, tissue injury, or excessive potassium intake. Decreased serum potassium (hypokalemia) can be due to inadequate intake, gastrointestinal losses without replacement, movement of potassium into cells secondary to alkalosis (potassium enters cells as acidic protons exit) or insulin action (potassium enters cells with glucose), use of beta-adrenergic medications (induces insulin secretion and cellular potassium uptake), hypomagnesemia (decreases renal potassium reabsorption), hyperaldosteronism, or to renal loss from diuretic use. Markedly abnormal serum potassium concentrations can cause patients to experience gastrointestinal symptoms, weakness, and cardiac arrhythmias.

With hypokalemia, each 1 mEq/L decrease in serum potassium concentration requires 200 to 400 mEq replacement. Replacement should be oral if possible, but intravenous potassium can be given at 0.7 mEq/kg lean body weight over two hours (not exceeding 20 mEq/hr, although even this rate can be painful locally to veins). Hyperkalemia can be treated with furosemide (Lasix®), combined infusions of glucose and insulin, bicarbonate, correction of metabolic acidosis (if present), and calcium gluconate in the case of significant electrocardiograph (EKG) changes. In extreme cases, dialysis can be used. In chronic cases, oral sodium polystyrene sulfonate binds potassium and decreases gastrointestinal absorption.

FLUID VOLUME DEPLETION

Total body fluid volume may decrease due to dehydration, hemorrhage, gastrointestinal fluid losses, inadequate fluid replacement, or to sequestering of fluid in interstitial spaces as a response to trauma or inflammation ("third spacing," such as during surgery). Electrolyte concentrations often are normal when the loss of fluid is isotonic or because the kidneys compensate for the lack of volume. Weight loss, decreased skin turgor, and tachycardia may be evident. If volume loss is extreme, blood pressure, renal perfusion, and urine output decline. It is unfortunate to some degree that Mother Nature chose to redistribute blood flow away from the kidneys during hypotensive episodes, because without adequate renal perfusion, the kidneys cannot compensate by regulating electrolyte concentrations properly. Teleologically, a possible benefit of this may be to minimize further fluid loss by preventing kidneys from producing urine, but it comes at a cost of ischemic renal injury. Monitoring urine output is an indirect method of assessing vascular perfusion, because adequate perfusion tends to be associated with adequate urine output. The minimum amount of waste solute that the kidneys must excrete each day to maintain homeostasis is about 600 mEq. Maximal renal concentrating ability is approximately 1,200 mEq/L, therefore, approximately 500 mL of urine must be produced daily to effectively excrete metabolic wastes, a minimum of about 20 mL/hr mean urine output. Urine output less than this in an obstetric patient is due most often to inadequate renal perfusion and, if prolonged, may lead to renal ischemia and failure. To allow a margin of safety, 30 mL/hr is used commonly as the threshold for adequate urine output.

Table 2.3: Parenteral Fluid Electrolyte Composition (mEq/L)

Solution	Na	Cl	K	Ca	Mg	Other	Osmolality
Extracellular Fluid	142	103	4	5	3	27*	280 to 310
Lactated Ringer's	130	109	4	3		28†	273
Normal Saline 0.9%	154	154					308
D$_5$-1/2 Normal Saline	77	77					407
D$_5$W			50 grams glucose per liter				253

Modified from Shires, 2009.   *HCO$_3$- †Lactate

If the intravascular space is depleted, fluid replacement should be isotonic to the fluid lost. In obstetric patients, this usually means a salt (crystalloid) solution such as lactated Ringer's or 0.9% normal saline (Table 2.3). Lactated Ringer's contains several electrolytes in concentrations similar to serum. Normal saline (NS) contains isotonic sodium chloride in concentrations slightly above serum but contains no other electrolytes. Five percent dextrose in water (D$_5$W) is slightly hypotonic when infused, but the 50 gm/mL glucose is metabolized quickly in the body, leaving markedly hypotonic free water. Hypotonic solutions dilute the plasma, leading to extravasation of fluid into the interstitial space due to osmotic imbalance. Even with isotonic fluid (crystalloid), most fluid administered intravenously quickly equilibrates across blood vessel walls into the interstitium because there is no protein in crystalloid to maintain intravascular colloid osmotic pressure. This is why pre-epidural fluid boluses should be given just before epidural placement; the administered fluid does not stay in the intravascular space very long. A general rule for volume resuscitation of a hemorrhaging pregnant woman is to give three times as much crystalloid as the estimated blood loss, with the knowledge that most of this fluid will extravasate out of the vessels into the interstitium. Although colloid solutions such as albumin or fresh-frozen plasma can be given during volume resuscitation, they may not be available immediately, and proteins within these solutions may be metabolized to yield free water, so they usually are not recommended.

MAINTENANCE HYDRATION FOR HOSPITALIZED OBSTETRIC PATIENTS

Maintenance hydration is predicated on balancing fluid and salt losses. In a normal pregnant patient, 3,000 mL of intravenous water intake per day is reasonable, because it is not much more than normal adult intake, and translates into 125 mL/hr, which is one liter per eight-hour shift. Intake should include 50 to 90 mEq of sodium per day; by this criterion, D_5-1/2 normal saline (NS) provides plenty. Several days without potassium are tolerated easily by a patient with normal kidneys. If nothing is ingested by mouth for more than several days, however, potassium should be replaced by adding 20 mEq to each liter of intravenous crystalloid. If potassium is lost due to vomiting, emesis volume should be replaced mL for mL with NS plus 20 mEq/L KCl. Because potassium is concentrated intracellularly, moderate to severe potassium losses will lower serum potassium concentrations only 1 to 2 mEq/L, as potassium moves extracellularly to accommodate losses, but will require large volumes of potassium to replete intracellular stores (150 to 600 mEq). Potassium should not be infused faster than 20 mEq/hr, because it is caustic to veins and can cause cardiac arrhythmias.

VOLUME OVERLOAD IN OBSTETRIC PATIENTS

Volume overload in obstetric patients most often is due to overzealous administration of intravenous fluids. This may happen during hydration as an initial treatment for preterm labor. The theory is that with dehydration the pituitary gland secretes antidiuretic hormone (ADH) to conserve water, and ADH has an oxytocin-like effect that could stimulate uterine contractions. Whether or not this is a cause of preterm labor is debatable, but hydration does decrease ADH secretion as well as its uterotonic action. Although hydration is a common therapy for possible preterm labor or preterm uterine activity in the setting of dehydration, there is no evidence that true labor responds to hydration. When preterm labor is treated with tocolytics, beta-adrenergic drugs (e.g., terbutaline) can alter capillary permeability and further decrease intravascular COP. This predisposes the patient to pulmonary edema from transudation of fluid into the alveoli of the lungs. Overhydration exacerbates this. It is essential that the patient receiving tocolytics not receive excessive saline or lactated Ringer's solution, especially if urine output is suboptimal, because the combination of tocolytics and overhydration can cause pulmonary edema.

After an epidural anesthetic is administered, blockade of sympathetic nerves may cause vasodilation and a decline in perfusion. To avoid this, fluids usually are infused just before the epidural is placed. Because water and salts are freely permeable across capillary membranes, however, much of this fluid quickly leaks into the interstitial space. With this in mind, it is important to infuse the fluids as close to the time the epidural is placed as possible; otherwise, the benefits will be lost and the risk of overhydration is increased.

Fluid management of preeclampsia is controversial. Women with preeclampsia may be volume contracted, and it seems logical to hydrate them or even to give colloid to improve perfusion. This has not been shown to improve outcome but invites overhydration and pulmonary edema. Low urine output in preeclampsia may reflect volume contraction (in which case a fluid bolus may be helpful) or it may represent renal vasospasm, when plasma volume may be adequate but renal perfusion is low due to renal artery constriction. Giving extra fluid to a patient with renal artery constriction risks fluid overload. Unless invasive central hemodynamic monitoring is available to differentiate between the two entities, maintenance fluids should be infused at 100 to 125 mL/hr in an effort to maintain urine output at a minimum of 20 to 30 mL/hr. One or two fluid boluses of 500 mL can be infused over an hour if urine output is falling. If output does not improve, however, further administration of fluid should be avoided because this may lead to edema and pulmonary congestion. Central monitoring of serum or urine markers of fluid status may be indicated at this point to better direct management.

CONCLUSION

Pregnancy is a state of fluid loading due to many physiologic changes that are important to understand when making clinical management decisions. Vasodilation causes increased intravascular capacity and decreased peripheral resistance, resulting in increased Na^+ reabsorption and subsequent flow of water into the intravascular space. When intravascular volume increases, cardiac output also increases, optimizing perfusion of the uteroplacental unit. Homeostatic responses protect this increased circulatory blood volume even at the expense of aggravating other electrolyte disorders because of the critical importance of these cardiovascular adaptations to the developing pregnancy.

RELATED READINGS

1. Benedetti TJ and Carlson RW (1979). Studies of colloid osmotic pressure in pregnancy-induced hypertension. <u>American Journal of Obstetrics and Gynecology</u>, 135(3), 883-887.

2. Clark SL, Cotton DB, Pivarnik JM, Lee W, Hankins G, Benedetti T, and Phelan J (1991). Position change and central hemodynamic profile during normal third-trimester pregnant and postpartum. <u>American Journal of Obstetrics and Gynecology</u>, 164(3), 883-887.

3. Sambandam K and Vijayan A (2007). Fluid and electrolyte management (Chapter 3). IN: DH Cooper, AJ Krainik, SJ Lubner, and HEL Reno (Eds.), <u>Washington Manual of Medical Therapeutics</u> (Ed. 32), Philadelphia, PA: Lippincott Williams and Wilkins, 54-101.

4. Scorza WE and Scardella A (2010). Fluid and electrolyte balance (Chapter 6). IN: Belfort MA, Saade G, Foley MR, Phelan JP, and Dildy GA (Eds.), <u>Critical Care Obstetrics</u> (Ed. 5), Hoboken, NJ: Wiley-Blackwell, pp. 69-92.

5. Shires GT III (2015). Fluid and electrolyte management of the surgical patient (Chapter 3). IN: Brunicardi FC, Anderson DK, Billiar TR, Dunn DL, Hunter JG, Matthews JB, and RE Pollock (Eds.), <u>Schwartz's Principles of Surgery</u> (Ed. 10), New York, NY: McGraw-Hill, pp. 65-84.

Chapter 2 Review
Fluid Dynamics in Pregnancy

1. Colloid osmotic pressure is decreased during pregnancy. The intravascular proteins (albumin, fibrinogen, and globulin) are diluted by the increased water within the intravascular space. This causes less "pulling effect" and greater potential for fluid movement:

    A. into the venous system.
    B. out of the veins and into the glomeruli and collecting systems of the kidneys.
    C. into the interstitial space.

2. Select the correct statement(s) regarding hydration in obstetric patients.

    A. Volume overload most often is due to overaggressive administration of intravenous fluids.
    B. Secretion of antidiuretic hormone causes preterm labor.
    C. Hydration will halt true labor.
    D. Pulmonary fluid overload can result from overhydration.
    E. The treatment for low urine output in preeclamptic patients is serial rapid fluid boluses.
    F. The commonly accepted threshold for adequate urine output is 50 mL/hr.
    G. All of the above.
    H. B, C, E, and F only.
    I. A and D only.

3. The major solute responsible for osmotic "pull" in extracellular fluid is:

    A. potassium.
    B. calcium.
    C. sodium.
    D. oxygen.

4. Intravenous fluids bolused prior to regional anesthesia help to mitigate:

    A. the blockade of sympathetic nerves.
    B. the blockade of parasympathetic nerves.
    C. both A and B.
    D. neither A nor B.

5. In a normal adult, a typical hydration should be:

    A. 50 mL/hr.
    B. 100 mL/hr.
    C. 125 mL/hr.
    D. 200 mL/hr.

Chapter 2 Review Answers
Fluid Dynamics in Pregnancy

1. **The correct answer is** C. With the decrease in colloid osmotic pressure in the intravascular space, intravascular fluids are attracted to the higher colloid osmotic pressure present in the interstitial space.

2. **The correct answer is I.** Overhydration results in a further decrease in colloid osmotic pressure in the intravascular space resulting in an increase in fluid moving to the interstitial space and alveoli of the lungs.

3. **The correct answer is C.**

4. **The correct answer is A.** After an epidural anesthesia is administered, blockade of sympathetic nerves may cause vasodilation and a decline in perfusion. To avoid this, a bolus of intravenous fluid is infused.

5. **The correct answer is C.**

Chapter 3

Fetal Circulation and the Impact on Fetal Heart Rate Monitoring

INTRODUCTION

Assessing the health of the fetus is limited by our incomplete understanding of what represents normal human fetal activity, how the fetus adjusts to its unique environment, and what clinical signs indicate true fetal danger. Despite these limitations, building on what is known allows us to better understand why fetal heart rate (FHR) patterns look the way they do, and helps us to refine our interpretation of these patterns in light of what we know about fetal physiology.

FETAL CIRCULATION

The primary function of lungs is to oxygenate blood, and to this end, a person's lungs have the highest blood flow of any organ in the body. Although the fetus has lungs and practices breathing before delivery, all oxygen exchange occurs through the placenta, and, thus, fetal lungs require very little blood flow. Thin-walled fetal pulmonary vessels in the deflated lung are compressed to prevent high volumes of blood from entering the pulmonary circulation. If blood is forced into the fetal lungs over a prolonged period of time, the vessels respond by thickening their muscular walls to accommodate the increased pressures. Although this protects the fetal pulmonary vessels, the thickened vessel walls lead to pulmonary hypertension after birth, which leads to persistent fetal circulation and under-oxygenation of the neonatal blood. Because fetal circulatory needs are markedly different from that of the newborn's, fetal circulation itself is different, and a dramatic transition takes place at birth to reroute blood to the lungs. To understand this transition, one needs to understand fetal circulation.

The fetal-placental circulation is designed elegantly to provide well-oxygenated blood from the placenta to the brain, less-well-oxygenated blood to the rest of the body, and to move poorly oxygenated blood as quickly as possible back to the placenta. Between the placenta and brain exists a complex of liver, heart chambers, and lungs. How does the fetus preferentially route blood to certain organs, while maintaining the capacity to switch to a newborn circulation at birth in which its lungs, not the placenta, are the primary source of oxygen?

In the fetal circulation, oxygen derived from the mother's blood crosses the placental villi and is carried by the fetal red blood cells in the umbilical vein toward the heart (Figure 3.1). While some of this blood enters the liver, 25% bypasses the liver, passing through the ductus venosus (DV, a vessel connecting the umbilical vein to the inferior vena cava [IVC]) to join blood returning from the lower body. One might assume that the well-oxygenated DV blood and

Figure 3.1: Unique Adaptations of the Fetal Circulatory System.
Red indicates higher oxygenation, blue lower, and purple mixed oxygenation.

Ascending Aorta
Ductus Arteriosus
RA
LA
PA
Foramen Ovale
RV
LV
Ductus Venosus
Umbilical Vein
Descending Aorta
Placenta
Umbilical Arteries

RA: Right Atrium   RV: Right Ventricle
LA: Left Atrium   LV: Left Ventricle
PA: Pulmonary Artery

29

poorly oxygenated IVC blood would be mixed together and the PO$_2$ would average out. However, this is not the case. Because of the orientation of these two vessels, the well-oxygenated blood from the DV streams into the IVC with laminar (layered) flow. Although there is some mixing, a degree of oxygen gradient is maintained. As the blood enters the right atrium, most of the better-oxygenated blood preferentially flows across the foramen ovale (the canal between the right and left atria) directly into the left atrium. This blood then enters the left ventricle and is pumped out the aorta to supply the coronary arteries to the heart and the carotid arteries to the brain. The less well-oxygenated blood from the IVC mixes with poorly oxygenated blood from the superior vena cava and streams downward through the right atrium into the right ventricle and out the pulmonary artery.

As discussed earlier, if all of this blood now in the pulmonary artery (PA) passed upwards into the high-resistance lungs, the pulmonary vasculature would be overwhelmed and respond with muscular hypertrophy. To avoid this, there is a large shunt called the ductus arteriosus (DA, not to be confused with the DV by the liver) between the PA and the descending aorta. Blood pressure in the PA is relatively high because of the high pulmonary vascular resistance, whereas blood pressure in the aorta is relatively low due to the low-resistance placental shunt. This pressure gradient facilitates flow of fetal blood from the PA through the DA into the aorta, allowing most of the less-oxygenated blood to bypass the lungs and flow to structures in the lower body of the fetus, including some back to the placenta via the umbilical arteries originating from the fetal internal iliac arteries. The PO$_2$ in the umbilical arteries, therefore, represents the degree of oxygenation received by most fetal organs, although less than that received by the fetal brain. In this configuration, the right ventricle contributes the majority of the cardiac output and, therefore, is the dominant ventricle in fetal life. After delivery, the left ventricle takes this responsibility and becomes the ventricle primarily responsible for systemic circulation.

Distribution of Cardiac Output

Because the heart, brain, and adrenal glands are critical for fetal survival, these organs receive a significant proportion of the cardiac output. The kidneys, although vital for survival after birth, are not essential for immediate fetal survival because fetal waste filtration is handled by the placenta. For this reason, kidneys receive a lesser proportion of cardiac output than the brain, heart, and adrenals.

Cardiac Composition and Function

The fetal heart has a fundamentally different makeup and physiology from the adult heart. First, contractile elements make up only 30% of the myocardium of the fetal heart, compared to the adult heart myocardium, of which 60% is made up of contractile elements. Additionally, while the fetal heart can be stimulated to produce a heart rate up to 300 bpm and maintain cardiac output, cardiac output from the adult heart begins to decline above a heart rate of 170 to 180 bpm. For this reason, fetal tachycardias above 180 bpm are much better tolerated than this heart rate would be in an adult.

Neural Control of the Fetal Heart

Neural control of cardiac function represents a transitional process occurring late in gestation and continuing into the early newborn period. Parasympathetic innervation and function of the fetal heart is well developed by about 24 weeks' gestation. In contrast, while beta-adrenergic receptor function in the fetal heart is well developed, myocardial catecholamines are lower than in the adult and sympathetic innervation of the fetal heart is immature even late in gestation.

During this period in late gestation, beta-adrenergic receptor function in the fetal heart is influenced by bloodborne catecholamines from the fetal adrenal glands. As term approaches, catecholamines in the primary sympathetic nerve trunks of the fetal heart progress down to the terminal endings and begin to replace the adrenal hormones as the primary sympathetic contributor to normal fetal cardiac regulation.

Because of the differential timing of development of each of the important neural controlling systems in the fetus, the parasympathetic system dominates in fetal life. As a consequence, most of the cardiac responses observed in the fetus as it responds to insults such as hypoxemia or hemorrhage reflect stimulation of the parasympathetic system.

Energy utilization by the fetal heart is similar to that of the adult but the source of energy differs. In the fetus, carbohydrates such as glucose, pyruvate, and lactate provide most of the energy, while in the adult only 60% comes from carbohydrates with the rest from free fatty acids. These differences in energy sources, coupled with the increased fetal oxidative phosphorylation and increased electron transport activity reflecting cellular respiration in the mitochondria help explain why the fetal heart requires more myocardial blood flow per 100 grams of tissue than the adult.

FETAL BRAIN MATURATION AND FETAL CIRCULATION

From 24 weeks onward, the fetus exhibits two clearly defined patterns of fetal behavior: active sleep and quiet sleep. In active sleep, the fetus exhibits episodic breathing, sporadic movement, and increased FHR variability. In quiet sleep, the fetus decreases its breathing and movements, and FHR variability is reduced. These two behavioral states have a diurnal rhythm. Nonetheless, the normal term fetus oscillates between these two behavioral states every 20 or 30 minutes but occasionally up to one hour (Figure 3.2).

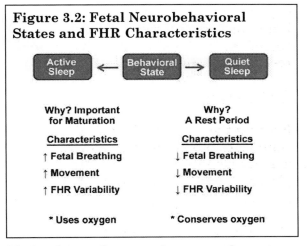

Figure 3.2: Fetal Neurobehavioral States and FHR Characteristics

What value to the fetus accrues from these changes in behavioral state? During active sleep, oxidative metabolism of the fetal brain increases. But why should the fetus alternate between these two very different behavioral states? From the psychology literature, we gain some insight into the answer. Following delivery, the newborn is exposed to tactile, auditory, and visual stimulation, all of which help the central nervous system mature. In fact, until a child is seven years old, and despite all of the visual, audio, and tactile stimulation it receives, his or her sensory centers still are maturing. But what type of intrauterine stimulation serves this purpose for the fetus? It seems that active sleep may be the global signal in the fetal brain that stimulates these centers to begin maturing prior to delivery; only when the fetus becomes a newborn does the outside world of sight, sound, and touch then take over. While active sleep is important for brain development, however, it is costly in terms of oxygen use. When the fetus is confronted by an episode of decreased oxygen availability, it will shift away from active sleep due to its oxygen expense.

Environmental Factors Affecting the Fetal Circulation

The fetus has considerable adaptive capabilities when confronted by a chronic reduction in oxygen delivery (Figure 3.3). When a pregnant woman has any condition that lessens placental oxygen delivery and produces mild-to-moderate hypoxemia, the fetus readjusts its activity to conserve energy. Even with moderate hypoxemia, absent such severe reductions that metabolic acidosis ensues, the fetus still can utilize its oxygen-dependent systems for generating cellular energy. In this scenario, the fetus transitions with into a quiet sleep behavioral state to conserve oxygen. The fetus reduces breathing motions, which eliminates energy expenditure by the diaphragm (a large muscle), and eliminates body rolls and motions of its extremities. Clinically, these changes are seen as decreased fetal activity, reduced breathing on ultrasound, and reduced baseline FHR variability during fetal monitoring. This degree of hypoxemia also may stimulate increased parasympathetic activity and late FHR decelerations. The fetus also can redirect its blood volume such that more oxygenated blood gets to the vital organs that it needs for survival (heart, brain, and adrenals). This preservation of vital organs is at the expense of other organs deemed less vital, such as the kidneys, to which blood flow is reduced. Reduced blood flow to the fetal kidneys means less glomerular filtration, which means less urine output, seen clinically as oligohydramnios. All of these compensatory actions by the fetus are components of assessment by FHR monitoring and biophysical profile (BPP), explaining why assessment of these characteristics allows evaluation of fetal health.

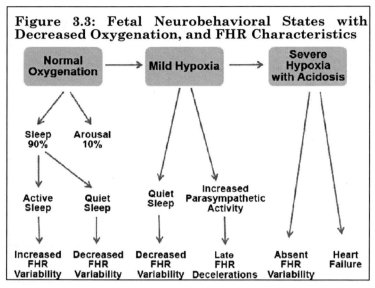

Figure 3.3: Fetal Neurobehavioral States with Decreased Oxygenation, and FHR Characteristics

TRANSITION TO NEWBORN CIRCULATION

Even though birth may seem a quick and abrupt event (Note: some laboring women may disagree), some of the biologic events that allow the fetus to transition to a newborn evolve over days and even weeks. At delivery, several significant events occur that allow the fetus, with its dependency on the placenta for oxygenation, to become an air-breathing newborn. These events involve eliminating the umbilical-placental circulation, closing the vascular shunts on which the fetus has relied, and ventilating the newborn lungs (Figure 3.4—next page).

After delivery, umbilical blood flow rapidly and spontaneously decreases to less than 20% of pre-delivery flow within 40 to 60 seconds due to vasoconstriction of both umbilical arteries and the umbilical vein. These changes, coupled with physically clamping the umbilical cord, abruptly remove what has been a low-resistance shunt, suddenly increasing systemic vascular resistance within the newborn and increasing arterial blood pressure. Delivery also subjects the newborn to immediate cold stress, which activates catecholamine release to produce an additional increase in the newborn's blood pressure and heart rate. This elevation in blood pressure reverses the right-to-left pressure gradient across the ductus arteriosus, directing blood back into the pulmonary circulation. More flow through the lungs means more pulmonary venous return to the left atrium. This increases left atrial pressure, reversing the pressure gradient between the right and left atria and causing the flap (septum primum) of the foramen ovale to push toward the left and close the passage.

Expansion of the lungs dramatically alters the pulmonary circulation. The unexpanded lungs of the fetus have high vascular resistance, but within the first several breaths, lung expansion by the neonate opens the pulmonary vessels, reduces the vascular resistance, and creates negative pressure within the chest allowing more blood to flow to the lungs. Decreased right-sided vascular resistance lowers right heart blood pressure, creating a further differential between the right and left heart, and helping to close the foramen ovale. Additionally, this acute expansion (as well as biochemical alterations in chloride and sodium transport) helps drive fluid from the lungs, which further increases pulmonary circulation. Within two hours, most alveolar fluid has been replaced by oxygen. With this, the alveoli transition from fluid secretion that was vital during fetal life, to fluid removal, making room for oxygen.

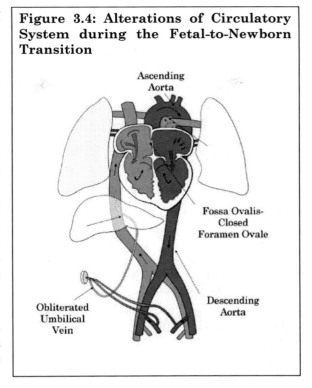

Figure 3.4: Alterations of Circulatory System during the Fetal-to-Newborn Transition

Ascending Aorta

Fossa Ovalis-Closed Foramen Ovale

Obliterated Umbilical Vein

Descending Aorta

Newborn respiration normally begins spontaneously within 15 seconds, resulting in a median oxygen saturation of 75% at one minute and 90% by three minutes. The change in oxygen saturation in the immediate newborn period also alters the caliber of the ductus arteriosus. In late fetal life, the DA is kept open by production of prostaglandin E_2 (PGE$_2$) in a reduced oxygen environment. With lung expansion, bradykinin is released which begins closure of the DA. As the oxygen saturation rapidly increases after birth, the enzymes responsible for producing PGE$_2$ are inhibited. As a result, PGE$_2$ production declines such that there is a 50% closure of the DA by 24 hours and 90% by 48 hours of life. In time, constriction of the DA leads to ductal wall ischemia and permanent closure.

CONCLUSION

In conclusion, the fetus is an amazing example of evolutionary adaptation. With its unique cardiovascular shunts to oxygenate critical organs during fetal life, its ability to change behavioral states to conserve oxygen when oxygen delivery is impaired, and its adaptation from placental oxygen dependency to self-sufficiency as an air-breathing organism following birth, fetal physiology is adapted uniquely to protect fetal health and prepare for independent living as a newborn.

RELATED READINGS

1. Adamson SL, Myatt L, and Byrne BMP (2011). Regulation of umbilical blood flow. (Chapter 74). IN: RA Polin, WW Fox, and SH Abman (Eds.), <u>Fetal and Neonatal Physiology</u>, (Ed. 4), Philadelphia, PA: Elsevier, Saunders, pp. 827-937.

2. Assali NS, Brinkman CR, Woods JR, Dandavino A, and Nuwayhid B (1977). Development of neurohumoral control of fetal, neonatal, and adult cardiovascular functions. <u>American Journal of Obstetrics and Gynecology</u>, 127:(7)748-759.

3. Boddy K, Dawes GS, and Fisher R (1974). Foetal respiratory movements, electrocortical and cardiovascular responses to hypoxemia and hypercapnia in sheep. <u>Journal of Physiology</u>, 243:599-618.

4. Clyman RI (2011). Mechanisms regulating closure of the ductus arteriosus. (Chapter 73). IN: RA Polin, WW Fox, and SH Abman (Eds.), <u>Fetal and Neonatal Physiology</u> (Ed. 4), Philadelphia, PA: Elsevier, Saunders, pp. 821-827.

5. Freed MD and Plauth WH Jr (1998). The pathology, pathophysiology, recognition and treatment of congenital heart disease. IN: RW Alexander, RC Schlant, and V Fuster (Eds.), <u>Hurst's The Heart</u> (Ed. 9), New York, NY: McGraw Hill, pp. 1925-1993.

6. Fineman JR and Clyman R (2009). Fetal Cardiovascular Physiology (Chapter 12). IN: RK Creasy, R Resnik, JD Iams, CJ Lockwood, and TR Moore (Eds.), <u>Creasy and Resnik's Maternal-Fetal Medicine</u> (Ed. 6), Philadelphia, PA: Elsevier, pp. 159-170.

7. Friedman WF (1973). The intrinsic physiologic properties of the developing heart. IN: WF Freidman, M Lesch, and EH Sonnenblick (Eds.), <u>Neonatal Heart Disease</u>, New York, NY: Grune and Stratton.

8. Richardson BS, Patrick JE, and Abduljabbar H (1985). Cerebral oxidative metabolism in the fetal lamb. Relationship to electrocortical state. <u>American Journal of Obstetrics and Gynecology</u>, 153:426-431.

9. Rudolph AM (2001). The fetal circulation and postnatal adaptations (Chapter 1). IN: AM Rudolph (Ed.), <u>Congenital Diseases of the Heart, Clinical-Physiological Considerations</u> (Ed. 3), Armonk, NY: Futura Publishing Company, pp. 3-44.

10. Schlant RC, Sonnenblick EH, and Katz AM (1998). Normal physiology of the cardiovascular system (Chapter 3). IN: RW Alexander, RC Schlant, and V Fuster (Eds.), <u>Hurst's The Heart</u> (Ed. 9), New York, NY: McGraw-Hill, 81-124.

Chapter 3 Review
Fetal Circulation and the Impact on Fetal Heart Rate Monitoring

1. The fetal circulation works in parallel, rather than in series like the adult circulation. Therefore, unlike the adult, the dominant ventricle for the fetus is the:

   A. right ventricle.
   B. left ventricle.

2. The fetal-placental circulation is designed to preferentially provide well-oxygenated blood from the placenta to the:

   A. brain, liver, and lungs.
   B. heart, liver, and lungs.
   C. brain, heart, and adrenal glands.
   D heart, lungs, and gastrointestinal tract.

3. The terms below all represent an active sleep or quiet sleep fetal behavioral state. Choose all that represent a quiet sleep behavioral state.

   A. Episodic breathing
   B. Reduced FHR baseline variability
   C. Increased FHR baseline variability
   D. Decreased breathing
   E. Decreased movements
   F. Sporadic movement

4. Which of the following are responsible for the fetus's transition to extrauterine life?

   A. The umbilical-placental circulation is eliminated.
   B. Clamping of the umbilical cord eliminates umbilical-placenta circulation and raises the blood pressure in the neonate's aorta.
   C. The flow across the ductus arteriosis is reversed.
   D. Catecholamine release increases the neonate's blood pressure and heart rate.
   E. Expansion of the neonate's lungs occurs.
   F. All of the above
   G. A, B, and C only
   H. D and E only

5. Fetal responses to mild hypoxia include:

   A. decreased quiet sleep.
   B. increased parasympathetic activity.
   C. increased motion.
   D. marked FHR variability.

Chapter 3 Review Answers
Fetal Circulation and the Impact on
Fetal Heart Rate Monitoring

1. **The correct answer is A.** During extrauterine life, the left ventricle contributes the majority of the cardiac output. During fetal circulation, the right ventricle is responsible for the majority of cardiac output.

2. **The correct answer is C.** The heart, brain, and adrenal glands are vital to the fetus for survival.

3. **The correct answers are B, D, and E.**

4. **The correct answer is F.**

5. **The correct answer is B.** When moderate hypoxemia occurs in the fetus, the fetus will transition to a quiet behavioral state to conserve oxygen. In addition, there is increased parasympathetic activity and late FHR decelerations will occur during contractions.

Chapter 4

Fetal Oxygen and Acid-Base Metabolism

INTRODUCTION

The rationale for antepartum or intrapartum fetal assessment of "fetal well-being" requires an understanding of oxygen delivery to the fetus, as well as of the fetal responses to compromised oxygen delivery and subsequent acid-base changes. Early investigators compared partial pressures of oxygen (PO_2) from women and their fetuses' umbilical cord blood and noted a disparity between maternal PO_2 in the upper-90s and fetal PO_2 in the mid-20s. They initially concluded that the fetus must exist in a hypoxic environment (i.e., one deficient in oxygen). With improved understanding of the fetal physiology, however, we now understand that the normal fetus is not hypoxic and, through a number of adaptive mechanisms, delivers oxygen to its cells in the same efficient way as an adult. This chapter will discuss how oxygen is conveyed from mother to fetus, how acid-base balance is maintained, and what happens when this system goes awry.

HEMOGLOBIN

Hemoglobin is a tetramer (made up of four units), consisting of two pairs of different proteins, the major ones being α (alpha), ß (beta), γ (gamma), and ε (epsilon). These proteins are similar in length but differ in their exact amino acid sequences, differences that change their oxygen binding characteristics. The two primary hemoglobins are adult hemoglobin ($α_2β_2$, also called hemoglobin A or HgA) and fetal hemoglobin ($α_2γ_2$, hemoglobin F or HgF).

The basic unit consists of a central heme molecule of four pyrrole rings linked in a planar circle (Figure 4.1). This complex unit contains many conjugated double bonds and appears deep red due to its ability to absorb light at the low end of the visible spectrum when oxygen is bound. One atom of iron (ferrous iron, Fe^{2+}) is at the center of this circular arrangement.

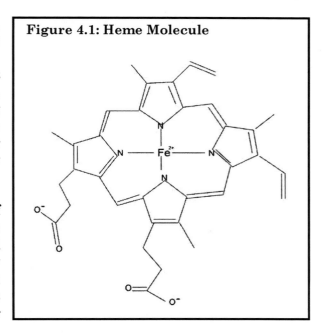

Figure 4.1: Heme Molecule

OXYGEN AND ADULT HEMOGLOBIN

Oxygen is transported either dissolved in plasma or bound to hemoglobin. Because oxygen dissolves poorly in plasma (it dissolves poorly in water overall), 98% of it is bound to hemoglobin. Adult hemoglobin can bind four oxygen molecules, one for each pyrrole ring. Oxygenation of hemoglobin is accompanied by a structural change in hemoglobin's configuration: when one oxygen molecule is bound, some of the double bonds are ruptured. While this may sound harmful, it actually is beneficial because conformational changes following each bond rupture makes it easier to bind additional oxygen (referred to as *cooperative binding kinetics*). This allows oxygen to bind easily when oxygen is plentiful (e.g., in the pulmonary capillaries), with cooperative binding helping to quickly saturate hemoglobin. Conversely, this also helps release oxygen at the less-oxygen-rich tissue level. With release of each oxygen molecule to the cells, the double bonds reform, loosening heme's hold on the remaining oxygen molecules and facilitating their release too.

FETAL HEMOGLOBIN

Like HgA, HgF consists of two alpha chains, but the ß (beta) chains have been replaced by 2 γ (gamma) chains. This makes the structure of HgF ($\alpha_2\gamma_2$) instead of ($\alpha_2\beta_2$) as in HgA. The biggest functional difference is that gamma chains in HgF do not bind 2,3-diphosphoglyceric acid (DPG, discussed in the next section) such that in low oxygen stages, HgF retains a higher affinity for oxygen than does HgA. This means that at the placenta, where maternal and fetal circulations meet, the HgF has a higher affinity than maternal hemoglobin for oxygen. This allows the fetus to easily extract oxygen from maternal hemoglobin, since HgF will bind oxygen avidly and carry high volumes of bound oxygen to the fetal cells despite the seemingly low PO_2 of fetal blood.

This difference in oxygen affinity between types of hemoglobin is measured by determining the "P50" level, or the partial pressure of oxygen that half-saturates hemoglobin. Adult hemoglobin has a P50 of 26 mmHg, meaning that at a PO_2 of 26 mmHg, 50% of the HgA will be saturated. Fetal hemoglobin has a lower P50 of 20 mmHg, meaning that it takes less oxygen tension to reach this same degree of saturation in the fetus than it does in an adult (Figure 4.2). In the third trimester, the fetus gradually begins to shift to HgA. By a few weeks after birth, the infant will have replaced HgF completely.

Figure 4.2: Oxygen Saturation Curve for Maternal and Fetal Hemoglobin

OXYGEN SATURATION CURVE FOR MATERNAL AND FETAL HEMOGLOBIN

HgF

Maternal HgA

INCREASING O₂ SATURATION

INCREASING PO₂

Note that at the same oxygen tension (PO₂), fetal hemoglobin is much more saturated with oxygen than maternal hemoglobin.

FACTORS AFFECTING FETAL HEMOGLOBIN FUNCTION

The degree of oxygenation of fetal red blood cells (i.e., location on the oxygen saturation curve) is affected by the environment that the red blood cell (RBC) encounters, as depicted in Figure 4.3. Certain conditions, such as increased heat, lower pH (acidosis), and increased PCO_2—all waste products of cell metabolism—exist in the peripheral tissues and will swing the oxygen saturation curve to the right. With this change, the fetal RBC rapidly releases oxygen and takes on CO_2. By contrast, at the oxygen-rich placenta, where less heat, a higher pH, and lower PCO_2 exist, the oxygen saturation curve swings to the left, such that at the same PO_2, the fetal RBC will take on oxygen. Both of these shifts facilitate delivery of oxygen to the tissues and removal of CO_2 waste.

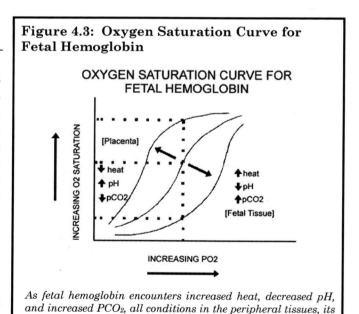

Figure 4.3: Oxygen Saturation Curve for Fetal Hemoglobin

OXYGEN SATURATION CURVE FOR FETAL HEMOGLOBIN

INCREASING O2 SATURATION

[Placenta]

↓ heat
↑ pH
↓ pCO2

↑ heat
↓ pH
↑ pCO2

[Fetal Tissue]

INCREASING PO2

As fetal hemoglobin encounters increased heat, decreased pH, and increased PCO₂, all conditions in the peripheral tissues, its oxygen dissociation curve swings to the right and oxygen is released. At the placenta, the opposite conditions (decreased heat, increased pH, and decreased PCO₂) lead to a swing in the oxygen dissociation curve to the left and more oxygen is taken up.

2,3-DIPHOSPHOGLYCERIC ACID (2,3-DPG OR DPG)

Another mechanism affecting hemoglobin's oxygen-carrying capacity involves the production and hemoglobin's binding of 2,3-diphosphoglyceric acid (2,3-DPG or DPG for short, also called 2,3-BPG). Cellular metabolism requires oxygen, and a metabolic product of glucose breakdown is DPG. In peripheral tissues, where oxygen and glucose are actively utilized, levels of DPG are high. DPG binds to partially oxygenated hemoglobin, further reducing oxygen affinity and causing it to release remaining oxygen more easily. This also means that DPG causes hemoglobin to bind oxygen less avidly, which would seem counterproductive in the lung. This is not a problem, however, because PO_2 is high in the lungs, and DPG tends to be displaced from hemoglobin by oxygen, increasing hemoglobin's oxygen uptake as a result. Thus, the system is balanced nicely to facilitate oxygen uptake in the lung and release in the periphery.

2,3-diphosphoglyceric acid decreases oxygen-binding avidity, but because of structural differences between the beta (adult) and gamma (fetal) chains, HgF (alpha$_2$-gamma$_2$) does not bind 2,3-DPG. Therefore, HgF binds oxygen more avidly than does adult hemoglobin. This lack of 2,3-DPG binding, in conjunction with the high maternal-fetal transplacental oxygen gradient, allows the fetus to extract oxygen from the mother readily. High fetal cardiac output circulates the blood quickly to the periphery, where the reversed oxygen gradient and environmental conditions (decreased pH, increased PCO_2, and increased heat) result in release of oxygen to the tissues.

OXYGEN TRANSPORTATION

Oxygen is used to metabolize glucose into water and carbon dioxide (CO_2), and produce abundant energy in the form of adenosine triphosphate (ATP) to fuel cell functions. In the absence of oxygen, glucose is metabolized anaerobically. The anaerobic process is inefficient, however, producing less ATP and generating lactate and other organic (non-carbonic) acids.

Inhaled air is a mixture of several gases including nitrogen, oxygen, and CO_2. Because these gases consist of molecules in a state of random motion, the molecules that make up each gas exert a pressure that is caused by molecular collisions. The total pressure of a gas mixture is the sum of the partial pressures exerted by each gas. Different gases exert different relative pressures because each is influenced by the number and type of molecules making up the gas and by the temperature. Therefore, the *partial pressure of oxygen*, or PO_2, is understood best not as an absolute measure of quantity, but as a measure of gradient and driving force. If there are more free molecules of a gas on one side of a space than on the other side, the partial pressure will be higher on that first side, and net flow will be toward the side with fewer molecules until the partial pressure are equal. In biologic terms, this is the force driving oxygen into the blood or, alternatively, how much pressure it takes to keep a given volume of oxygen dissolved.

Oxygen dissolves poorly in water, the major constituent of blood. While increasing PO_2 (e.g., administering higher concentrations of oxygen) will drive more oxygen into water, the additional volume dissolved will not increase nearly as dramatically as the increase in PO_2. However, if molecules with high oxygen avidity are added to the water (e.g., hemoglobin as in blood), they will bind oxygen in addition to that amount dissolved, the net result being much more oxygen absorbed at a given PO_2. The actual volume of oxygen that enters blood is proportional to a combination of its partial pressure, the solubility of oxygen in water, the oxygen binding avidity of molecules in the blood, and the temperature of the blood. *Oxygen capacity* defines the maximum amount of oxygen that can be carried by a unit of blood. The proportion of maximal oxygen-carrying capacity achieved is referred to as *oxygen saturation* and depends on the partial pressure of oxygen to which the blood is exposed and the combination of chains that make up the hemoglobin. Thus, high or low PO_2 only correlates with volume of dissolved oxygen when comparing two solutions with the same oxygen-binding capacity and temperature.

OXYGEN DELIVERY AT THE PLACENTAL LEVEL

Fetal oxygenation begins at the placenta. Well-oxygenated maternal blood from terminal branches of the uterine arteries enters the intervillous space into which dip the placental villi containing fetal capillaries. Maternal blood initially flows out at the top of the space and moves slowly downward along the villi, eventually draining via the uterine veins. During this process, oxygen passes across the villus membranes from the maternal to the fetal circulations, with the maternal oxygen concentration gradually decreasing, fetal oxygen content increasing, and the gradient between the two nearly equalizing. By the time maternal blood has made its way down the entire cone of fetal capillaries, its PO_2 levels may exceed that of the fetal blood only by a few mmHg. Conversely, final PO_2 of fetal blood leaving the placenta is similar to that of maternal venous blood. The drive for this exchange is the gradient (difference in partial pressures) between maternal and fetal PO_2; the higher maternal PO_2 favors passage to the lower-PO_2 fetal blood, and the high-affinity fetal hemoglobin readily binds the transferred oxygen such that the fetal PO_2 remains relatively low despite the volume of oxygen transferred.

FETAL ELIMINATION OF METABOLIC BY-PRODUCTS

Carbon dioxide is one of the major byproducts of cell metabolism. Like oxygen, CO_2 moves across membranes by simple diffusion. Hemoglobin is capable of binding CO_2 directly when oxygen is released, and about 15% of the CO_2 carried in blood is bound to hemoglobin. Unlike oxygen, CO_2 is very soluble in water, and the volume of CO_2 dissolved in plasma is 20 times greater than that of oxygen. Because partial pressure of a gas determines the amount dissolved in plasma, and because most CO_2 is transported in the dissolved form, partial pressure is a more direct measure of plasma CO_2 content than it is of oxygen content.

To understand the role of CO_2, knowledge of how acids and bases interact is crucial. A proton is a part of an atom that has a positive charge, while an electron carries a negative charge. A hydrogen atom, with one proton and one electron, is neutral electrically. Remove the electron and the hydrogen atom becomes a single positive proton (H^+). Why is this important? An *acid* is a molecule with a weak attraction for protons (i.e., positively charged), while a *base* is a molecule with a strong attraction for protons (i.e., negatively charged). This means that acids easily release protons while bases actively bind them. Therefore, for the most part, the presence of free protons makes a solution acidic.

Catalyzed by carbonic anhydrase in RBCs, dissolved CO_2 reacts with H_2O to form carbonic acid (H_2CO_3), which rapidly dissociates into the proton H^+ and the base, bicarbonate (HCO_3^-). While a small amount of HCO_3^- is produced in plasma, most is produced from CO_2 in RBCs, which then diffuses out into plasma. Therefore, the main form of CO_2 transported in blood is HCO_3^-.

FETAL ACID-BASE BALANCE

The fetus metabolizes glucose and fatty acids to form CO_2, which can be converted into carbonic acid. As mentioned in the preceding paragraph, carbonic acid is balanced electronically but dissociates by losing a hydrogen proton (H^+) and becoming a negatively charged base, bicarbonate.

Bicarbonate can reenter the fetal RBC and combine with H^+ to form carbonic acid which then changes back into CO_2 and H_2O (Figure 4.4). This CO_2 rapidly crosses the placenta to enter the maternal circulation, removing it from the fetal compartment and allowing the pregnant woman to breathe it out through her lungs. The fetus also generates non-carbonic acids by anaerobic metabolism, such as uric acid from amino acids, and by incomplete combustion of carbohydrates and fatty acids, leading to the production of lactic acid and ketoacids. Unlike CO_2, these non-carbonic acids diffuse very slowly from the fetal to the maternal circulation.

Figure 4.4: Carbonic Acid and Metabolism

- $C_6H_{12}O_6$ (glucose) $+ 6\ O_2 \longrightarrow 6\ O_2 + 6\ H_2O$

- $CO_2 + H_2O \longleftrightarrow H_2CO_3$ (carbonic acid) $\longleftrightarrow H^+ + HCO_3^-$

Acid-base balance is measured by pH, the negative logarithm of the hydrogen ion concentration. Without going further into the math, a low pH implies an acid (more protons), while a high pH is consistent with a base (fewer protons). The fetus must prevent wide swings in pH, and does so by controlling the production of H^+ as well as using plasma bicarbonate (HCO_3^-) as a first-line buffer. Buffers absorb or release protons to maintain pH in a narrow range. Erythrocyte bicarbonate, inorganic phosphates, and charged plasma proteins all aid in buffering, especially when plasma bicarbonate systems are overwhelmed. On the other hand, when excessive bicarbonate is generated, it can associate with sodium (Na^+) to form sodium bicarbonate ($NaHCO_3$), preventing the blood from becoming overly alkaline. In this way, the concentration of individual types of molecules can control the direction of other reactions to maintain acid-base balance.

UNDERSTANDING BASE EXCESS

Of the many confusing concepts in acid-base balance, the term "base excess" (BE) is near the top of the list. Most of the body's buffers are bases that bind protons and, as such, a certain amount of "buffer base" must be available to maintain pH balance. If cells produce excessive volumes of acids that "use up" the buffer bases, then the amount of available base decreases. In some laboratories this is expressed as a calculated positive number indicating the degree of "base deficit." Although this makes intuitive sense, most laboratories use the alternative concept of "base excess," a negative number that denotes a "negative excess" (i.e., a deficit). In this construct, the more negative the base excess, the less buffer base is available, presumably because it has been used up buffering organic acids. Base deficit or excess is understood most easily as a measure of degree of metabolic acidosis (see below).

TYPES OF ACIDOSIS

There are two types of acidosis: respiratory and metabolic. Respiratory acidosis occurs when accumulation of CO_2 leads to proton release via carbonic acid formation. Although respiratory acidosis can be severe, acute cases are rapidly reversible as CO_2 is removed quickly, thus reversing the process and bringing pH back to normal. Short episodes of decreased oxygen delivery will cause a respiratory acidosis, but if the episodes resolve quickly, they usually are well tolerated and do not result in injury or in a change in base buffer levels. In these cases, the one-minute Apgar score may be low, but the five-minute score usually is normal. With respiratory acidosis, PCO_2 levels rise and pH falls, but base excess will be unchanged.

Metabolic acidosis in obstetrics, on the other hand, most often results from prolonged lack of oxygen. With metabolic acidosis, the cellular oxygen concentration is so low that normal energy/ATP production by glycolysis and the Krebs cycle cannot be maintained, so the cells switch to less-efficient anaerobic metabolism. This generates some energy but also many organic acids (such as lactic acid) that dissociate and release protons, further acidifying the blood. At delivery, the organic (or "fixed") acids are reflected in the umbilical arterial blood gas analyses by a low pH and bicarbonate, with an increasingly negative base excess (a "lack of excess base," i.e., too much organic acid, also called a base deficit in some laboratories).

Keywords for Understanding Acidosis

Acidosis:	Increase in hydrogen ions in tissue
Acidemia:	Increase in hydrogen ions in blood
Hypoxia:	Reduced oxygen content in tissue
Hypoxemia:	Reduced oxygen content in blood
Metabolic acidosis (pure):	Usually normal PCO_2; low HCO_3^-; overly negative base excess
Respiratory acidosis (pure):	High PCO_2; HCO_3^- acutely elevated but would normalize over time if chronic; normal base excess
Mixed acidosis:	High PCO_2; low HCO_3^-; overly negative base excess

Unfortunately, prolonged anaerobic metabolism will not satisfy the cells' energy needs for very long, and eventually, the cells "run out of gas," sustain injury, and then may die. Equally unfortunate is that, unlike acute respiratory acidosis in which the retained CO_2 can be blown off quickly and normal pH rapidly restored as soon as umbilical cord flow is restored or the baby is delivered, organic acids are not metabolized quickly, nor do the cells rapidly reverse their metabolism to resume aerobic energy production as soon as oxygen again is made available. Because of this, metabolic acidosis persists longer and has a much stronger association with hypoxic organ damage. This is the infant with low one- <u>and</u> five-minute Apgar scores, who, in the worst case, requires intensive resuscitation (see below) and may show evidence of neurologic or multiorgan dysfunction after birth.

CAUSES OF ACIDOSIS

Acute respiratory acidosis results from any condition that impairs transport of CO_2 from fetus to mother (e.g., umbilical cord compression, uterine tachysystole compressing the uterine arteries, initial response to placental abruption, or maternal hypoventilation). For example, if umbilical cord compression impairs CO_2 diffusion from fetus to mother, fetal CO_2 accumulates and more carbonic acid is formed. Carbonic acid, in turn, dissociates into bicarbonate and hydrogen ions (H^+), thus making the blood acidic. If umbilical cord compression is released, flow is restored, CO_2 passes back across the placenta, PCO_2 returns to normal, the acidosis rapidly reverses, and usually, there is full recovery. If umbilical cord compression is not released, or released only for a short time, however, the persistent lack of umbilical cord flow and resultant lack of oxygen delivery to the fetus eventually will cause frank hypoxia, a switch to anaerobic metabolism, the generation of lactic acid, and a metabolic acidosis. The risk of fetal injury rises with duration and severity of oxygen deprivation.

Unlike respiratory acidosis, there are many possible causes of metabolic acidosis, including anything causing persistent, severe, uteroplacental compromise (e.g., extensive placental abruption or infarction, prolonged umbilical cord prolapse, persistent tachysystole, etc.), certain rare metabolic diseases due to inherited enzyme defects, or maternal conditions such as renal failure, chronic severe diarrhea, alcoholism, or diabetic ketoacidosis. In obstetrics, however, fetal metabolic acidosis almost always means that there has been a period of decreased oxygenation.

UMBILICAL BLOOD GAS ASSESSMENT

Compression of uterine arteries by myometrial contractions during labor briefly decreases utero-placental blood flow, causing transient declines in maternal-fetal gas exchange. As such, normal labor creates a degree of metabolic stress and, therefore, results in mild decreases in fetal pH, PO_2, and bicarbonate, and a slightly more-negative base excess, all without long-term consequences. Fortunately, the high degree of reserve in a normal placenta prevents this from causing fetal injury.

Table 4.1: Mean Umbilical Cord Blood Gas Values (Mean ± SD)

	Artery	Vein
pH	7.24 ± 0.07	7.32 ± 0.06
PCO₂ (mmHg)	56 ± 9	44 ± 7
PO₂ (mmHg)	18 ± 7	29 ± 7
BE (mEq/L)	-4 ± 3	-3 ± 2

Modified from Thorp (1989)

The question of whether umbilical artery and vein blood gas values should be assessed routinely immediately after delivery is an ongoing debate. Umbilical artery (UA) blood best reflects fetal status because it represents central arterial blood flowing from the fetal aorta through the iliac arteries into the UA. Umbilical vein blood best reflects placental function in that the vein contains blood that just passed through the placenta. Because the umbilical vein blood has just received oxygen and given off CO_2, its values almost always look "better" than the artery's (presuming that the placenta is functional). Normal values are depicted in Table 4.1, and the most common indications for obtaining cord pHs are listed in Table 4.2.

Table 4.2 Common Indications for Fetal Blood Gas Sampling

> - Operative or cesarean delivery for fetal compromise
> - Low (less than 7) five-minute Apgar score
> - Fetal growth restriction
> - Category II or III fetal heart rate tracing
> - Maternal metabolic or systemic disease
> - Intrapartum fever or chorioamnionitis
> - Multifetal gestation
> - Known or suspected fetal anomaly or disorder
> - Preterm delivery
> - Meconium

PREDICTIVE VALUE OF UMBILICAL BLOOD GASES

Nearly 100% of vigorous newborns and 80% of "depressed" infants will have normal blood gas values. Apgar scores correlate poorly with neonatal hypoxic injury. Fetal pH determinations correlate better, although the majority of infants born even with a pH less than 7.0 will be normal (especially if the acidosis was pure respiratory). Because low Apgar scores and "neonatal depression" may be confused with "birth asphyxia" (especially in preterm neonates, in whom Apgar scores may be low due exclusively to prematurity), obtaining UA blood gas values can be helpful in ruling out hypoxia and acidosis as causes of the depression. A reasonable approach at or near term is to clamp and cut a segment of cord promptly at delivery. If Apgar scores are greater than 6 at one and five minutes, UA blood gas values likely do not need to be requested. If Apgar scores (especially at five minutes) are less than 7, it may be prudent to send UA blood in a heparinized syringe for blood gas analysis. Once the cord segment is clamped, even delays of up to 60 minutes will not affect the blood gas values unduly.

A normal umbilical cord blood pH rules out acute birth asphyxia (although not necessarily some past asphyctic episode). A low pH, high PCO_2, and normal BE represent a pure respiratory acidosis, usually carrying an excellent prognosis. These babies often have a low one-minute but normal five-minute Apgar score as they breathe off retained CO_2 immediately after delivery. A low pH and BE more negative than -8 indicate some degree of metabolic acidosis, regardless of the PCO_2.

As with respiratory acidosis, these babies often have low one-minute Apgar scores, but because of the longer duration of hypoxia and delayed resolution of metabolic acidosis, they also may have low five-minute Apgar scores. Although most such babies also do well, the risk of neurologic injury is higher than with a pure respiratory acidosis. Overall, umbilical cord blood gas analysis not only assesses the degree of acidosis (if any), but often also sheds light on the underlying pathophysiology that led to it. A normal UV blood gas panel is consistent with normal placental function; fetal hypoxia in those circumstances implies an umbilical cord complication. Most cases of abnormal UV gas panel imply impairment of uteroplacental function (placental abruption, maternal hypotension, placental infarction, infection, etc.)

CONCLUSION

At times, learning about normal and abnormal fetal blood-gas biology may seem valuable only as an academic exercise. Not so! Understanding the concepts of fetal oxygenation and acid-base balance underlies our understanding of antenatal and intrapartum fetal monitoring, and of relating neonatal conditions at birth to umbilical artery blood gas results. In addition, an understanding of how the fetus compensates during periods of reduced oxygen-availability has contributed to the development of antepartum tests for fetal surveillance. It also demonstrates the specialized adaptations and capabilities of the fetus to allow survival in the intrauterine world.

RELATED READINGS

1. American College of Obstetricians and Gynecologists (2006). Committee Opinion #348: Umbilical cord blood gas and acid-base analysis. <u>Obstetrics and Gynecology</u>, 108(5):1319-1322.

2. Armstrong L and Stenson BJ (2007). Use of umbilical cord blood gas analysis in the assessment of the newborn. <u>Archives of Disease in Childhood: Fetal & Neonatal Edition</u>, 92(6):F430-434.

3. Duerbeck NB, Chaffin DG, and Seeds JW (1992). A practiced approach to umbilical artery pH and blood gas determination. <u>Obstetrics and Gynecology</u>, 79:959-762.

4. Guyton AC and Hall JE (2011). Transport of oxygen and carbon dioxide in blood and tissue fluids (Chapter 40). <u>Textbook of Medical Physiology</u> (Ed. 12), Philadelphia, PA: W.B. Saunders Company, pp. 495-504.

5. Meschia G (2014). Placental respiratory gas exchange and fetal oxygenation (Chapter 14). IN: RK Creasy, R Resnik, JD Iams, CJ Lockwood, TR Moore, MF and Greene (Eds.), <u>Creasy and Resnik's Maternal-Fetal Medicine: Principles and Practice</u> (Ed. 7), Philadelphia, PA: W.B. Saunders Company, pp. 163-174.

6. Nageotte MP (2014). Intrapartum fetal surveillance (Chapter 33). IN: RK Creasy, R Resnik, JD Iams, CJ Lockwood, TR Moore, and MF Greene (Eds.), <u>Creasy and Resnik's Maternal-Fetal Medicine: Principles and Practice</u> (Ed. 7), Philadelphia, PA: W.B. Saunders Company, pp. 488-506.

7. Thorp JA, Sampson JE, Parisi VM, and Creasy RK (1989). Routine umbilical cord blood gas determinations? <u>American Journal of Obstetrics and Gynecology</u>, 161(3):600-605.

Chapter 4 Review
Fetal Oxygen and Acid-Base Metabolism

1. The degree of oxygenation of fetal red blood cells is affected by the environment that the red blood cells encounter. Which of the following conditions will increase the oxygen demand of the fetus?

    A. Increased temperature
    B. Higher pH
    C. Increased carbon dioxide
    D. All of the above
    E. A and C only

2. Match the term in Column A with the definition in Column B.

Column A	Column B
1. Acidosis	A. Increased PCO_2, decreased HCO_3^-
2. Acidemia	B. Reduced oxygen content in the blood
3. Hypoxia	C. Normal PCO_2, decreased HCO_3^-
4. Hypoxemia	D. Increase in hydrogen ions in tissue
5. Metabolic acidosis	E. Increased PCO_2, HCO_3^- normal
6. Respiratory acidosis	F. Increase in hydrogen ions in blood
7. Mixed acidosis	G. Reduced oxygen content in the tissues

3. Which of the following is a normal umbilical artery blood gas profile?

    A. pH 7.40, PO_2 95 mmHg, PCO_2 35 mmHg
    B. pH 7.45, PO_2 80 mmHg, PCO_2 42 mmHg
    C. pH 7.30, PO_2 25 mmHg, PCO_2 52 mmHg
    D. pH 7.04, PO_2 23 mmHg, PCO_2 64 mmHg

4. Umbilical artery blood gas values are as follows: pH 7.15, PCO_2 70 mmHg, PO_2 20 mmHg, HCO_3^- 25 mEq/L, and the base excess -4 mEq/L. These values are indicative of:

    A. metabolic acidosis.
    B. respiratory acidosis.
    C. mixed respiratory and metabolic acidosis.
    D. normal umbilical artery cord blood values.

5. In low oxygen states:

    A. fetal hemoglobin has a higher affinity for oxygen than adult hemoglobin.
    B. fetal hemoglobin has a lower affinity for oxygen than adult hemoglobin.

Chapter 4 Review Answers
Fetal Oxygen and Acid-Base Metabolism

1. **The correct answer is E.** When there is increased body temperature, lower pH, and increased carbon dioxide levels, the fetus will release oxygen quicker, thereby resulting in an increased need for more oxygen.

2. **The correct answers are: 1-D, 2-F, 3-G, 4-B, 5-C, 6-E, 7-A.**

3. **The correct answer is C.**

4. **The correct answer is B.** Even though the pH is low and the PCO_2 is elevated, the PO_2, HCO_3^-, and the base excess are normal. This result indicates a respiratory acidosis, which will resolve quickly after birth with proper care.

5. **The correct answer is A.** The gamma chains in the fetal hemoglobin increase the affinity of the fetal hemoglobin for oxygen. This allows for a more rapid extraction from the maternal hemoglobin.

Chapter 5

Amniotic Fluid Physiology

INTRODUCTION

Amniotic fluid serves many purposes during pregnancy. It provides room for movement, is a protective cushion for the fetus and the umbilical cord, equally distributes warmth, serves as a destination for fetal urine (or meconium), has antibacterial properties, and is required at key stages for proper lung development. Normal amniotic fluid volume implies normal renal perfusion. Extremes of amniotic fluid volume, on the other hand, are associated with increased perinatal morbidity and mortality, for reasons that will be discussed below. Various methods using ultrasound allow for estimation of amniotic fluid volume (AFV), and this is incorporated into the process of antenatal fetal assessment.

COMPOSITION OF AMNIOTIC FLUID

The amniotic sac that contains the developing embryo forms in the fourth week of gestation. There are several sources for amniotic fluid production. As the pregnancy progresses through the first trimester, the amniotic fluid within this sac essentially is a transudate of fetal plasma through the thin, unkeratinized fetal skin and umbilical cord. Between 20 to 24 weeks' gestation, the composition of the amniotic fluid changes as the fetal skin becomes progressively more keratinized and impermeable. Contributions from fetal urine, lung secretions, and swallowing increase (Table 5.1) such that after 18 to 20 weeks' gestation, fetal urine is the principle source of amniotic fluid.

Table 5.1: Composition of Amniotic Fluid

Electrolytes:	Sodium and osmolality fall progressively throughout gestation, while urea and creatinine increase.
Proteins:	Total protein levels peak in the late second trimester, with levels 1/10 that of fetal plasma.
Lipids:	Increasing lecithin (lung surfactant) in the third trimester reflects lung maturity.
Bilirubin:	Bilirubin decreases progressively in the third trimester, reflecting decreased red blood cell breakdown and increased metabolism of breakdown products.
Cells:	Fetal cells from the skin and bladder may be used for karyotyping.
Antibacterial factors:	Lysozymes, peroxidases, interferons—alpha and beta—all appear in the amniotic fluid.
Antioxidants:	Vitamin C is concentrated preferentially and may provide protection from oxidant damage (e.g., infection).

AMNIOTIC FLUID VOLUME REGULATION

The amount of amniotic fluid present at any one time reflects the balance between production (fetal urination and lung secretions) and removal (fetal swallowing and fluid resorption through the fetal surface of the placenta). Production and removal are balanced (Table 5.2—next page), and reach their peak at approximately one liter in the third trimester (around 34 weeks' gestation). Although the amniotic fluid may seem a static pool, proper balance entails that the entire volume be re-circulated daily. In fact, some investigators have noted even higher circulation rates and estimate that this turnover occurs several times every 24 hours.

Amniotic fluid in the second and third trimester is derived almost exclusively from two sources: the lung from secretions and the kidney in the form of urine. As the fetal renal system matures in the second and third trimesters, rates of urination progressively increase five- to ten-fold relative to the first and early-second trimesters. In times of fetal stress (further discussed in the section "Oligohydramnios" below), changes in the fetal circulation that result in decreased blood flow to the fetal kidneys may cause a significant decrease in urination and, subsequently, lead to low AFV, or oligohydramnios. Fetal lung secretions are very similar to fetal plasma, and their unimpeded release is vital to normal lung development. During labor, increased production of catecholamines and antidiuretic hormone increase pulmonary sodium absorption and decrease lung fluid secretion, allowing the lungs to "dry out" and prepare the fetus's transition to air breathing. Lack of these physiologic labor-related changes increases the risk of neonatal "wet lung" (also known as transient tachypnea of the newborn) in infants delivered by cesarean section before labor.

Table 5.2: Amniotic Fluid Balance in the Term Pregnancy

Flow into Amniotic Cavity **(1,000 mL per day)**	Flow out of Amniotic Cavity **(1,000 mL per day)**
Fetal urine (800 mL)	Fetal swallowing (600 mL)
Lung secretions (200 mL)	Transplacental flow (400 mL)

The principle route of amniotic fluid resorption is through fetal swallowing. The fetus is able to swallow fluid early in the second trimester, with the amount swallowed steadily increasing as the gestation proceeds. By term, nearly 600 mL of fluid is swallowed each day by the fetus. Inhibition of fetal swallowing due to upper gastrointestinal tract obstruction or neuromuscular abnormalities (e.g., cleft lip, oral tumors, esophageal atresia, certain neurologic conditions, etc.) will then lead to excess amniotic fluid, or polyhydramnios, which can increase the risks of preterm labor or preterm rupture of membranes. Finally, fluid resorption through surface vessels on the fetal side of the placenta allows transfer of fluid from the amniotic cavity back to the fetus.

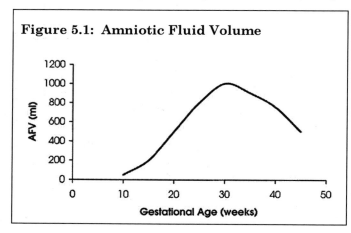

Figure 5.1: Amniotic Fluid Volume

The amount of amniotic fluid increases throughout the pregnancy until early in the third trimester, when it measures approximately one liter (Figure 5.1). After that time, the level stabilizes for a short time until near term when it slowly decreases.

EVALUATION OF AMNIOTIC FLUID VOLUME

Ultrasound is the most common method to quantify AFV, although the "gold standard" for research is the dye-dilution technique in which a known quantity of dye is injected into the amniotic sac, allowed to disperse, and a sample aspirated and the dye concentration determined. Back-calculating allows accurate determination of amniotic fluid volume. For obvious reasons, however, this technique is not very practical for clinical use, and much to the relief of pregnant women, various sonographic techniques allow us to approximate AFV. There is a relatively good association between the subjective assessment of amniotic fluid volume by a trained sonographer and the semi-quantitative techniques of the maximum vertical pocket or the amniotic fluid index (AFI). There is debate as to which technique is most accurate; some support AFI while others prefer the single-deepest pocket technique. In multiple gestations, the DVP is used to approximate AFV. The single-deepest-pocket is fairly self-explanatory: the maximal vertical depth of amniotic fluid volume that one can measure. The AFI is measured by adding the depth of the single deepest fluid pocket in each of the four quadrants of the uterus, as defined by the maternal umbilicus, while keeping the ultrasound transducer in the sagittal plane and perpendicular to the floor. The measured pocket(s) should not contain fetal parts or loops of umbilical cord.

DISORDERS OF AMNIOTIC FLUID VOLUME

Abnormalities in amniotic fluid volume can lead to a number of pregnancy related complications. In some pregnancies, there may be too much amniotic fluid or too little. When there is too much amniotic fluid, this is called polyhydramnios, and when too little, oligohydramnios. Either may be a sign of a complication or, in itself, lead to a complication. Because AFI varies with gestational age (Figure 5.1—previous page), normative curves have been established to determine when these thresholds are reached. Although the exact thresholds for decreased AFV (oligohydramnios) are controversial, available data from randomized control trials support the use of the deepest vertical pocket of amniotic fluid volume of 2 cm or less to diagnose oligohydramnios. The diagnostic criteria for polyhydramnios also are controversial. However, according to the Society of Maternal Fetal Medicine Consult Series, if the amniotic fluid index is 24 cm or more, or a single vertical pocket is over 8 cm, amniotic fluid is increased (polyhydramnios).

Polyhydramnios

Polyhydramnios occurs in approximately 1% to 2% of pregnancies for a variety of reasons (see Table 5.3). Most of the time, the amount of excess fluid is mild, occurs in the last trimester of pregnancy, and for the majority of cases a diagnosis cannot be found. These are called idiopathic polyhydramnios. In these cases, significant pregnancy complications are rare and the prognosis is excellent. It also can be associated with large fetuses (macrosomia) or maternal diabetes. The association with diabetes is theorized to be due to a fetal osmotic diuresis in an effort to excrete excess glucose, although there is little experimental evidence supporting this. Aneuploidy and hydrops for any reason can present as polyhydramnios, and persistent polyhydramnios in the absence of a known etiology should lead to consideration of genetic

Table 5.3: Selected Causes of Polyhydramnios

> Macrosomia (with or without maternal diabetes)

> Diabetes mellitus

> Fetal central nervous system anomalies (anencephaly, spina bifida, hydrocephaly)

> Fetal gastrointestinal anomalies (esophageal atresia, duodenal atresia, gastroschisis, omphalocele)

> Fetal chest mass (pleural effusion, diaphragmatic hernia)

> Chromosomal anomalies or genetic syndromes

amniocentesis. More severe polyhydramnios results when the fetus is unable to swallow adequately or absorb normal amounts of amniotic fluid secondary to anomalies of the brain or digestive tract. Subsequent over-distention of the uterine cavity by the excess fluid then increases the risk for preterm labor, premature rupture of the membranes, umbilical cord prolapse, malpresentation, and placental abruption.

Evaluation and Management of Polyhydramnios

The evaluation of polyhydramnios includes a sonographic anatomic survey to rule out structural anomalies or hydrops, review of maternal glucose testing, and consideration of fetal karyotyping. Regular assessment of presentation may reveal breech position or transverse lie. Because of the risk of umbilical cord prolapse, some patients with polyhydramnios are admitted for induction of labor in a controlled setting, rather than risk spontaneous rupture of membranes at home. This may be more important when the cervix is several centimeters dilated and the head is not well applied before labor has begun.

Oligohydramnios

Oligohydramnios complicates approximately 10% of all pregnancies. It can occur at any time, although it most commonly is noted in the third trimester and particularly is common in post-term pregnancies. The degree of oligohydramnios generally depends on the underlying causative process (Table 5.4). Before term, premature rupture of the membranes is a common cause, along with uteroplacental insufficiency.

Maternal/placental cardiovascular disease can lead to decreased placental perfusion, leading to fetal hypoxemia and, redistribution of fetal blood flow to the brain, heart, and adrenal glands, and away from the kidneys, with a subsequent decline in

Table 5.4: Selected Causes of Oligohydramnios

> Premature rupture of membranes

> Uteroplacental insufficiency

> Fetal genitourinary anomalies (renal agenesis, bladder outlet obstruction, renal dysplasia)

> Post-term pregnancy

> Chromosomal problems or genetic syndromes

fetal urine production. Past the due date, AFV tends to decrease, possibly as the placenta nears the end of its programmed lifespan.

Substantial decreases in amniotic fluid also may occur when there is urinary tract obstruction or failure of the kidney to develop (renal agenesis). In these cases, normal amniotic fluid from diffusion across the placenta is present until 18 to 20 weeks' gestation, after which severe oligohydramnios develops. In cases where oligohydramnios is severe and prolonged over the key 18- to 22-week period of pulmonary alveolar development, there is a high risk of lethal pulmonary hypoplasia. Lack of amniotic fluid can also lead to musculoskeletal contractures and deformations. In addition, oligohydramnios can lead to the compression of a vulnerable umbilical cord, which can compromise fetal oxygenation and, if severe enough, lead to fetal demise.

Evaluation and Management of Oligohydramnios

The three immediate assessments following a finding of oligohydramnios are an estimate of fetal weight/growth, sonographic evaluation of the fetal urinary tract, and a speculum examination to rule out ruptured membranes. If growth is poor, umbilical artery Doppler and nonstress testing can help assess placental function, and a decision made regarding need for delivery. If membranes are ruptured, then expectant management until about 34 weeks is an option in the absence of labor or infection. In a preterm pregnancy with "idiopathic" oligohydramnios, twice-weekly nonstress tests and weekly AFV assessments usually can safely prolong gestational age until term.

CONCLUSION

Amniotic fluid is essential to proper fetal lung and musculoskeletal growth and development. Disorders in amniotic fluid volume require further detailed evaluation of mother and fetus, as they may be a marker of serious maternal or fetal disease. Ultrasound assessment of amniotic fluid volume provides useful information in the management of complicated pregnancies.

RELATED READINGS

1. American College of Obstetricians and Gynecologists (2014). Antepartum fetal surveillance. Practice Bulletin No. 145. <u>Obstetrics and Gynecology</u>, 124:182-192.

2. Beall M and Ross M (2008). Amniotic fluid dynamics (Chapter 3). IN: RK Creasy, R Resnik, and JD Iams (Eds.) <u>Creasy and Resnik's Maternal-Fetal Medicine: Principles and Practice</u> (Ed. 6), Philadelphia, PA: W.B. Saunders, pp. 47-54.

3. Callen PW (2007). Amniotic fluid: Its role in fetal health and disease (Chapter 20). IN: <u>Ultrasonography in Obstetrics and Gynecology</u> (Ed. 4), Philadelphia, PA: W.B. Saunders, pp. 758-779.

4. Dashe JS, Pressman EK, and Hibbard JU (2018). SMFM Consult Series #46: Evaluation and management of polyhydramnios. <u>American Journal of Obstetrics and Gynecology</u>, 219 (4): B2-B8.

5. Harman CR (2008). Assessment of fetal health (Chapter 21). IN: RK Creasy, R Resnik, and JD Iams (Eds.) <u>Creasy and Resnik's Maternal-Fetal Medicine: Principles and Practice</u> (Ed. 6), Philadelphia, PA: W.B. Saunders, pp. 361-396.

6. Gilbert WM (2007). Amniotic fluid disorders (Chapter 31). IN: SG Gabbe, JR Niebyl, and JL Simpson (Eds.) <u>Obstetrics: Normal and Problem Pregnancies,</u> (Ed. 5), Philadelphia, PA: Churchill Livinstone Elsevier, pp. 834-845.

7. Reddy UM, Abuhamad AZ, Levine D, Saade GR, Fetal imaging invited participants. Fetal Imaging: executive summary of a joint Eunice Kennedy Shriver National Institute of Child Health and Human Development, Society for Maternal Fetal Medicine, American Institute of Ultrasound in Medicine, American College of Obstetricians and Gynecologists, American College of Radiology, Society for Pediatric Radiology, and Society of Radiologists in Ultrasound (2014). Fetal Imaging Workup. <u>Obstetrics and Gynecology</u>, 123(5):1070-1082.

Chapter 5 Review
Amniotic Fluid Physiology

1. In the first trimester of pregnancy, amniotic fluid primarily is made up of:

    A. fetal urine.
    B. maternal urine.
    C   transudate of fetal plasma.

2. True or False. After 18 to 20 weeks' gestation, fetal urine is the principle source of amniotic fluid.

    A. True
    B. False

3. At its peak, in the third trimester, amniotic fluid volume should be:

    A. one liter.
    B. two liters.
    C. three liters.
    D. five liters.

4. Select the correct statement regarding amniotic fluid volume.

    A. Ultrasound is not useful in measuring amniotic fluid volume.
    B. The amniotic fluid index (AFI) is measured by adding the depth of the single deepest fluid pocket in each of the four quadrants of the uterus.
    C. Amniotic fluid volume is the same through a normal pregnancy.
    D. An AFI of greater than 10 cm is considered polyhydramnios.

5. When an amniotic fluid index is performed by ultrasound, the diagnosis of low amniotic fluid is made when amniotic fluid measures:

    A. less than 5 cm.
    B. 10 cm.
    C. 20 cm.

Chapter 5 Review Answers
Amniotic Fluid Physiology

1.   The correct answer is C.

2.   The correct answer is A.

3.   The correct answer is A.

4.   The correct answer is B.

5.   The correct answer is A.

Chapter 6

Assessment of Uterine Activity

INTRODUCTION

Monitoring fetal heart rates (FHR) requires monitoring of the uterine activity as well, particularly in the presence of FHR decelerations. Benign, early FHR decelerations and potentially ominous, late FHR decelerations can look surprisingly alike, and it generally requires a concurrent tracing of uterine contractions to determine which is which. In addition, the FHR may respond to prolonged contractions, tachysystole, or coupling, such that an understanding of uterine activity, how it is measured, what is normal and what is not, and how it can affect FHR patterns is a key element of FHR monitoring.

NORMAL UTERINE ACTIVITY

Although there is not unanimous agreement among experts as to the specific parameters of "normal uterine activity," the significant characteristics of uterine activity have been described as follows:

- Average normal uterine resting tone is 8 to 12 mmHg.

- The *frequency* of contractions reflects the time interval between the beginning of one contraction and the beginning of the next. It often is referred to as the number of contractions observed in a ten-minute interval, averaged over 30 minutes. Contractions every two to three minutes are considered normal during labor. Any contraction-mediated decrease in uteroplacental perfusion is alleviated during the one- to two-minute interval between contractions, allowing the fetal PO_2 to normalize.

- Contraction *intensity* is the magnitude of the intrauterine pressure above the baseline uterine resting tone. With an intrauterine pressure transducer, an "adequate" contraction generally is 40 to 60 mmHg at the peak of the contraction, although intensities up to 100 mmHg are not uncommon. Intensity of the contraction also can be assessed by palpation as mild, moderate, or strong. Because of normal placental reserve, most contractions are tolerated by a healthy fetus, regardless of whether the intensity peaks at 40 or 100 mmHg.

- The *duration* of the contraction is the length of time in seconds from the beginning to the end of one contraction (50 to 70 seconds is average). This can be determined by palpation or by monitor, although an external monitor may undercount the duration, depending on where it is placed on the uterus.

Because contractions cause a repetitive pressure on the maternal-placental-fetal unit and, as such, constitute a brief "stress," they are useful for analysis of the fetal heart response. A contraction may affect the fetus by compressing the umbilical cord between the fetal body and uterine wall, altering the exchange of nutrients and oxygen/carbon dioxide at the uteroplacental interface, or by pressing the fetal head against the maternal pelvis in the latter half of labor. All of these situations may influence the FHR by giving rise to periodic (contraction-related) changes in FHR or decelerations (see also Chapter 7 on decelerations).

Tocodynamometry

Uterine contractions can be monitored externally with a pressure transducer known as a tocodynamometer. The tocodynamometer is placed on the maternal abdomen, usually over the uterine fundus. As the uterus contracts, the tocodynamometer detects the change in abdominal excursion and contour, displaying it as a contraction on the external fetal monitoring strip. External monitoring allows for accurate assessment of the frequency of contractions but cannot assess the resting uterine tone or absolute strength of contractions, because it does not measure intrauterine pressure. Additionally, how well the external monitor measures the exact onset and resolution of contractions also is influenced by placement of the belts and the maternal habitus. If difficulty is encountered, the frequency and duration of uterine contractions also may be assessed by palpation.

Intrauterine Pressure Catheter

Intrauterine pressure catheter (IUPC) monitoring involves inserting a catheter through the cervix into the amniotic cavity to monitor the strength of uterine contractions. For placement, the amniotic membranes must be ruptured. Unlike the tocodynamometer, which only provides a record of the frequency of uterine contractions, the IUPC provides a clear recording of the frequency, baseline tone, and peak contraction strength (Figure 6.1). The value of the IUPC, when compared with the external tocodynamometer, is that it allows for a more accurate assessment of uterine contractions and, when oxytocin is being used, titration of the dose. Another advantage of the IUPC is that it can function as an access port for amnioinfusion.

Figure 6.1: FHR tracing before and after the placement of an IUPC showing the difference in appearance and assessment options between the two monitoring options

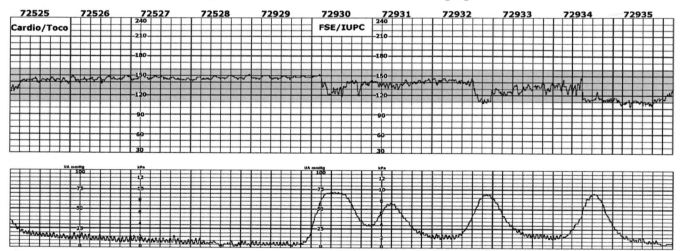

Limitations of the IUPC include the following:

- Rupture of amniotic membranes and adequate cervical dilation are required.

- The procedure is invasive.

- Risk of infection and uterine perforation may be increased.

- Careful attention to technique, especially when zeroing and calibrating, is required for accurate data.

- The catheter tip or pressure transducer may become wedged against a fetal part, preventing the production of a pressure curve or producing a distorted, damped, or truncated pressure wave.

- Intrauterine pressure catheters should be used with caution with certain types of infections and conditions (e.g., human immunodeficiency virus, hepatitis C, or significant vaginal bleeding of unknown etiology).

Uterine Activity Monitoring

The primary uses of IUPCs are either to correlate FHR changes with contractions or to assess the adequacy of labor. When labor is not progressing well, it is essential to be able to time and assess contraction intensity to determine whether labor should be augmented. If contractions are less frequent than three or four per ten minutes, or of weak intensity, this likely is dysfunctional labor, and, in the absence of cephalopelvic disproportion, labor augmentation should be considered to improve the quality and frequency of contractions. If contractions can be monitored externally and palpated, an IUPC is not necessary to make this determination, but if the frequency and intensity of contractions is uncertain (such as when the patient is obese), an IUPC can provide much more accurate information to guide management. If the IUPC records contractions as every two to three minutes and of normal intensity, oxytocin is <u>not</u> indicated even when the cervix is not dilating, because one risks tachysystole, the uterus with its attendant risks of fetal compromise, and even uterine rupture. The goal of augmentation is achievement of normal labor patterns.

An advantage of an IUPC is the ability to characterize unusual contraction patterns that may not be appreciated as well by a tocodynamometer. Elevated uterine baseline tone is difficult to assess externally. Generally, it remains at or below 20 mmHg, allowing resumption of uteroplacental blood flow between contractions. When the baseline is persistently elevated, placental perfusion may be affected. Although some baseline tone elevations may be artifacts, and others well-tolerated by the fetus, when oxytocin is being used (a common reason for elevated tone), the clinician should consider whether the dose should be decreased, whether the IUPC needs to be replaced or recalibrated, or whether the patient's position should be changed.

Figure 6.2: Tachysystole. Note associated late FHR decelerations.

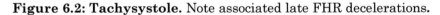

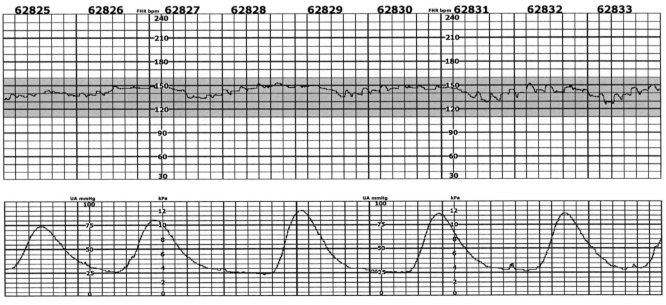

Another pattern seen clearly with an IUPC is tachysystole (Figure 6.2—previous page). Tachysystole is a pattern of rapid contractions defined as greater than five uterine contractions within ten minutes, averaged over a 30-minute window. Tachysystole should always be qualified as to the presence or absence of associated FHR decelerations.

Tachysystole can be seen in spontaneous contractions as well as in prostaglandin- or oxytocin-stimulated labor. Management differs depending on whether contractions are spontaneous or stimulated. When spontaneous, contractions tend to be low intensity, sometimes called "irritability." Uterine abruption should be ruled out and hydration should be considered. When tachysystole follows pharmacologic stimulation, the recommendation is to decrease or stop the oxytocin infusion or remove the prostaglandin, consider hydration, and if there are concerning FHR features (e.g., late or prolonged FHR decelerations), consider temporary administration of a tocolytic such as a dose of terbutaline.

Through the use of an IUPC, FHR patterns can be correlated more accurately with the timing and strength of contractions. This facilitates FHR interpretation, allowing obstetric providers to initiate appropriate interventions and then to determine the fetus's response to the intervention.

INTRAPARTUM AMNIOINFUSION

The technique of intrapartum amnioinfusion was first described in 1983. Since that time, there have been numerous controlled, prospective reports on its use. Oligohydramnios is the most common indication for amnioinfusion in the published studies, followed the presence of variable FHR decelerations. For variable decelerations, the concept is that restoring intra-amniotic fluid may provide a cushion for a compressed umbilical cord, although this would be less likely if fluid volume is normal. Ruptured amniotic membranes are a prerequisite for intrapartum amnioinfusion, of course, and by definition, fluid volume after membrane rupture will be less than it was before rupture, making it plausible to assume some decrease in amniotic fluid volume in a labor complicated by recurrent variable FHR decelerations. The most common infusion protocol in a review of published trials begins with insertion of an IUPC, followed by a 500 mL bolus of sterile saline administered through the IUPC over approximately one hour, and then by a 150 mL/hr constant infusion (Table 6.1).

Table 6.1: Technique of Intrapartum Amnioinfusion

1. Used for variable FHR decelerations in the setting of suspected oligohydramnios, in the absence of repetitive late decelerations.
2. The amniotic membranes must be ruptured and the FHR continuously monitored.
3. Insert an IUPC.
4. Infuse a 500 mL bolus of sterile saline through the IUPC over 60 minutes, followed by a 150 mL/hr constant infusion.
5. Monitor the total volume infused, as well as the estimated volume passed per vagina.
6. Monitor intrauterine pressure every 15 to 30 minutes. Stop the infusion if the pressure rises above 25 mmHg.
7. If the fetal heart rate tracing worsens, further fetal evaluation or delivery should be undertaken.

The range of initial boluses in reported studies varies from 250 to 1,000 mL, and the maintenance infusion rates vary between 150 to 250 mL/hr. Lactated Ringer's solution occasionally has been used in place of saline. Some centers use infusion pumps to control the flow, as well as blood warmers to avoid infusing cool saline. It has not been shown that there is any advantage to using pumps or warmers, as long as the infusion rates are not excessive and the total infusion and return volume is monitored carefully.

Fetal monitoring should be performed during and following amnioinfusion, and intrauterine pressures should be maintained in the normal range. Uterine overdistention and iatrogenic polyhydramnios can cause excessive intrauterine pressures that may result in decreased uterine artery blood flow, decreased oxygen delivery to the placenta, and subsequently decreased fetal oxygenation. Infusion volumes can be monitored either by pad weights or ultrasonographic amniotic fluid volume determinations if there is a suggestion that fluid volumes are not balanced.

Effectiveness of Amnioinfusion

The majority of reports on intrapartum amnioinfusion have demonstrated reductions in the rates of cesarean delivery, concerning fetal status, and meconium below the vocal cords at delivery. Despite the decrease in these fetal outcome markers with amnioinfusion, the effect on low five-minute Apgar scores (less than 7) is inconsistent. Some authors have reported fewer low five-minute Apgar scores in patients receiving amnioinfusion when compared with similar patients who did not receive amnioinfusion, but others have reported an *increase* in the number of low five-minute Apgar scores in amnioinfusion patients. Similarly, the effect of amnioinfusion on postpartum endometritis is uncertain, with most studies reporting decreased incidences, but several reporting large increases. While an IUPC may introduce bacteria into the amniotic cavity, the flow of fluid may serve to "flush out" intrauterine bacteria.

Amnioinfusion for Meconium

Amnioinfusion, in the past, has been proposed as a way of diluting meconium and possibly decreasing the incidence of intrapartum meconium aspiration syndrome (MAS). It also is possible that amnioinfusion might replenish low amniotic fluid volume and alleviate umbilical cord compression, thereby restoring normal fetal oxygenation, raising umbilical artery pH, and minimizing in-utero fetal gasping. While amnioinfusion does decrease the incidence of meconium below the cords, there is no evidence that this translates into a lower risk of MAS. A recent large randomized trial by Fraser et al. reported no improvement in perinatal outcome for amnioinfusion done for meconium, and meconium no longer is considered an indication for amnioinfusion.

Disadvantages of Amnioinfusion

Disadvantages of amnioinfusion include the need for continuous fetal monitoring, inability of the pregnant woman to ambulate during and after infusion, and the 30- to 60-minute time course from the beginning of infusion until its effectiveness can be assessed. There are reports of rare complications such as umbilical cord prolapse, increased uterine tone leading to fetal hypoxia, maternal fluid overload, and amniotic fluid embolism. Amnioinfusion should not be undertaken to relieve persistent late FHR decelerations; such FHR decelerations imply uteroplacental insufficiency, for which amnioinfusion is not effective. Some consider chorioamnionitis to be a contraindication to amnioinfusion, although amnioinfusion has been proposed in patients with chorioamnionitis specifically for the purpose of administering intrauterine antibiotics—this remains a topic of controversy.

RELATED READINGS

1.   Association of Women's Health, Obstetric, and Neonatal Nurses (2015). Fetal Heart Rate Monitoring Principles and Practices (Ed. 5), Washington, D.C.: AWHONN.

2.   American College of Obstetricians and Gynecologists (2009). Induction of labor. ACOG Practice Bulletin #107.

3.   American College of Obstetricians and Gynecologists (2010). Management of intrapartum fetal heart rate tracings. ACOG Practice Bulletin #116.

4.   American Academy of Pediatrics, American College of Obstetricians and Gynecologists (2007). Guidelines for Perinatal Care (Ed. 6).

5.   Association of Women's Health, Obstetric, and Neonatal Nurses Practice Monograph (2009). Cervical Ripening and Induction and Augmentation of Labor.

6.   Freeman RK, Garite TJ, and Nageotte MP (2003). Instrumentation and artifact detection (Chapter 4). IN: Fetal Heart Rate Monitoring (Ed. 3), Baltimore, MD: Lippincott Williams & Wilkins, 36-53.

7.   Freeman RK, Garite TJ, and Nageotte MP (2003). Uterine contraction monitoring (Chapter 5). IN: Fetal Heart Rate Monitoring (Ed. 3), Baltimore, MD: Lippincott Williams & Wilkins, 54-62.

8.   Garite TJ (2017). Intrapartum fetal evaluation (Chapter 15). IN: SG Gabbe, JR Niebyl, JL Simpson, et. al (Eds.) Obstetrics: Normal and Problem Pregnancies (Ed. 7), Philadelphia, PA: Churchill Livingston.

9.   Macones GA, Hankins GDV, Spong CY, Hauth J, and Moore T (2008). The 2008 National Institute of Child Health and Human Development Workshop Report on Electronic Fetal Monitoring: Update on Definitions, Interpretation, and Research Guidelines. American College of Obstetricians and Gynecologists. 112:661-666.

10. Thorp JM (2018). Clinical aspects of normal and abnormal labor (Chapter 36). IN: R Resnik, CJ Lockwood, TR Moore, et.al. (Eds.) Creasy and Resnik's Maternal-Fetal Medicine: Principles and Practice (Ed. 8), Philadelphia, PA: Saunders Elsevier.

Chapter 6 Review
Assessment of Uterine Activity

1. Uterine activity is defined by:

    A. contraction frequency.
    B. contraction duration.
    C. relaxation between contractions.
    D. all of the above.
    E. A and B only.

2. Which of the following describes the relationship between uterine contractions and fetal status in labor?

    A. Contractions may affect maternal blood flow to and from the placenta.
    B. Duration of contractions, intensity, and relaxation intervals are equally as important as frequency of contractions.
    C. Fetal responses to contractions as seen in fetal heart rate tracings are interdependent and evolve over time.
    D. All of the above

3. True or False. In the presence of tachysystole, describing frequency of uterine contractions fulfills the requirement for adequate documentation.

    A. True
    B. False

4. Select the correct statement(s) regarding the assessment of uterine contractions.

    A. Contraction frequency alone is a complete assessment of uterine activity.
    B. Duration, intensity, frequency, and relaxation time between contractions are of equal importance.
    C. The presence or absence of FHR decelerations always should be assessed when tachysystole is suspected.
    D. The terms tachysystole, hyperstimulation, and hypercontractility may be used synonymously.
    E. Tachysystole applies to both spontaneous and stimulated labor.
    F. All of the above
    G. A and D only
    H. B, C, and E only

5. Amnioinfusion during labor requires:

    A. intact amniotic membranes.
    B. infusion of 500 mL/hr of sterile saline for a constant infusion until delivery occurs.
    C. monitoring of intrauterine pressure every 15 to 30 minutes.
    D. a resting uterine tone of 30 mmHg.

Chapter 6 Review Answers
Assessment of Uterine Activity

1. **The correct answer is D.**

2. **The correct answer is D.**

3. **The correct answer is B.** Uterine contractions also should be described with regard to duration, intensity, and relaxation time between contractions. In addition, fetal heart rate interpretation also should be documented.

4. **The correct answer is H.** The terms hyperstimulation and hypercontractility are not defined by the National Institute of Child Health and Human Development and should be abandoned. The full assessment contains more than just frequency of contractions.

5. **The correct answer is C.**

Chapter 7

Fetal Heart Rate Monitoring: Technology, Baseline, and Variability

EXTERNAL FETAL MONITORING TECHNOLOGY

Before addressing the elements of fetal monitoring, it is helpful to understand the capabilities and limitations of the technology we employ to detect and record fetal heart rate (FHR) patterns. An external cardiotachometer is a Doppler ultrasound device that transmits and receives ultrasound signals. The frequency of an ultrasound wave changes when there is movement of the tissues from which it reflects, a change referred to as a Doppler shift. When the Doppler is directed toward the fetal heart, cardiac motion creates Doppler shifts that the monitor detects and converts to an electronic signal. This signal is used as a marker of the fetal heartbeat, as well as to generate an audible sound produced by the monitor. The monitor is not a microphone "listening to the beating fetal heart," it is producing an artificial sound that results from the frequency changes caused by reflection of the ultrasound waves that are produced by a moving heart.

Because each Doppler wave lacks the triggering point characteristic of the R-wave of the electrocardiograph (ECG) signal, data are sampled along the waveform and superimposed upon subsequent waveforms, each of which also is sampled. Through autocorrelation, the monitor attempts to identify a recurring pattern among the accompanying noise within the waveforms (fetal or maternal movement, bowel motion, artifact, etc.), thereby enabling a reasonable estimate of heart rate. Depending on the age and make of the monitor, two or more waveforms may be sampled to produce this estimate.

Because this process involves a computerized "educated best guess" at what passes for a cardiac cycle, it is not 100% accurate. Also, and depending on the age of the monitor, there is a degree of averaging among adjacent beats, smoothing the tracing slightly. This may interfere with the precision of FHR recording and particularly is important regarding assessment of variability (see below). As autocorrelation algorithms have improved over the years, however, precision of external FHR monitoring has improved as well. The advantages of external FHR monitoring are that it is noninvasive and usually adequate; the disadvantages are that it may be impossible to obtain a satisfactory FHR tracing (e.g., extreme obesity or a very active fetus), may record maternal heart rate instead of fetal, can be difficult with multiple gestations, and some information may be lost through autocorrelation.

In recent years, external fetal ECG monitors have been developed. Currently, only approved by the FDA for external monitoring in obese patients, these monitors may overcome some of the issues described above.

FETAL SCALP ELECTRODE

If the external monitor is not tracing well, and the patient has ruptured amniotic membranes and is committed to delivery, a fetal scalp electrode (FSE) can be applied (literally piercing the surface of the fetal skin). This detects electrical signals as an internal fetal ECG, using the R-wave of the QRS complex as its reference for determining FHR. If functioning properly, an FSE gives a more accurate representation of FHR and variability, may circumvent artifacts from fetal and maternal movement, and avoids "The Belt" used to hold the monitor in place. Its disadvantages include being more invasive, occasional contraindications (e.g., an HIV-infected mother), the potential for misplacement (e.g., on an unappreciated face presentation), and the fact that it only can be used when the amniotic membranes are ruptured, the mother is committed to labor, and the cervix is dilated enough to apply the electrode.

Similar to autocorrelation, there is a logic function in the fetal monitor's microprocessor that attempts to filter out artifacts by rejecting signals coming at unexpectedly rapid or slow intervals (i.e., that are excessively different from one another). Without this logic function, considerable "noise" would be recorded on the fetal tracing. The logic always is functional when external (Doppler) cardiotachometers are used. This may result in the monitor eliminating and not recording actual "excessive" FHR changes such as those that occur with some fetal arrhythmias (Figure 7.1). With some brands of monitors, the logic is also functional when the internal scalp electrode is being used. Other monitors have a switch that permits the logic to be turned off when the internal direct-fetal ECG (scalp electrode) monitor mode is in use. Turning off the logic function when using the FSE (internal) mode results in the monitor's counting of the intervals between each successive R-wave of the fetal QRS complex, including those that vary excessively from the previous R-wave. This often is the case with frequent fetal premature atrial contractions, and may give rise to a signal that appears spikey with multiple vertical lines interrupting the tracing (Figure 7.1)

Figure 7.1

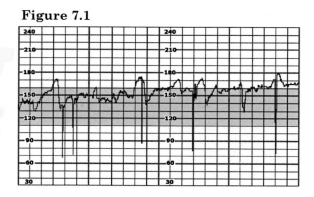

While the logic function usually works well, it can create problems when there are fetal heart arrhythmias. With very rapid heart rates, it may reject every other beat (they seem closer together than the microprocessor expects), halving the true rate. For analogous reasons, it may erroneously double slow rates. This is less problematic with FSE monitoring, but still can occur with extreme FHRs.

One might ask why the FSE does not detect the maternal ECG as well as the fetal ECG. Because of proximity, the fetal signal normally is stronger than the maternal signal, but because the strength of fetal signals can vary from one fetus to another, the monitor is programmed to search for the strongest signal, gradually lowering its threshold until it finds it. This is important in the case of a fetal demise, in which the threshold may be lowered so much in an attempt to find the nonexistent fetal heart signal that the maternal ECG is detected and displayed as if it were fetal, leading the unwary obstetric attendant to mistake the maternal "FHR" reading for that of a live fetus. Emergency cesarean sections have been done for fetal heart rate bradycardia only to deliver a macerated stillborn in whom death clearly occurred days before.

BASELINE FETAL HEART RATE

"Baseline" refers to the average FHR over a ten-minute period, rounded to the nearest 5 bpm, and not including episodic or periodic changes (i.e., accelerations or decelerations), periods of marked variability, or dramatic changes of 25 bpm or more during that ten minutes. At least two minutes of discernible baseline (not necessarily continuous) must be present during this ten-minute period. Normal baseline ranges from 110 bpm to 160 bpm. Baseline rates that are lower or higher than this for at least ten minutes are termed bradycardia or tachycardia, respectively. A normal baseline FHR is one of many indicators that fetal oxygen status is more likely to be adequate.

Baseline FHR tachycardia is defined as an FHR greater than 160 bpm persisting for at least ten minutes (again, excluding accelerations and decelerations) (Figure 7.2). Fetal tachycardia results from an increase in sympathetic and/or a decrease in parasympathetic autonomic nervous system tone, and often is associated with decreased variability (especially when the rate is above 180 bpm).

Sometimes a lengthy acceleration can be confused with baseline tachycardia. Continued observation usually resolves the question: if the heart rate stays high, it's tachycardia. If it declines to a previous baseline, it was a prolonged acceleration. Although baseline FHR is known to decrease as gestational age advances, the average difference from 28 weeks' gestation to term is only about 10 bpm. While premature fetuses may have slightly higher baseline FHRs than term fetuses, significant fetal tachycardia seldom can be attributed to prematurity alone. It requires evaluation for maternal or fetal factors that may increase the FHR (Table 7.1).

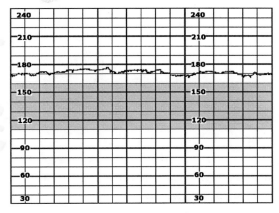

Figure 7.2: Fetal Tachycardia—FHR Greater Than 160 bpm for Greater Than or Equal to Ten Minutes

When the FHR exceeds 240 bpm, even a direct fetal ECG will not measure every consecutive R-wave interval. If the intervals between consecutive R-waves are less than 250 milliseconds (which corresponds to a rate of 240 bpm), the time is too brief for the monitor to process each R-wave. This may result in the monitor halving (e.g., recording 120 bpm for an actual rate of 240 bpm) or not recording an interpretable tracing. Fetal heart rates greater than 240 bpm may be seen with supraventricular tachycardia (SVT), paroxysmal atrial tachycardia (PAT), atrial fibrillation, or atrial flutter.

Table 7.1: Causes of Baseline FHR Tachycardia

Maternal	Fetal

➤ Fever/infection
➤ Dehydration
➤ Hyperthyroidism
➤ Anxiety
➤ Cigarette smoking
➤ Medication or drug response, e.g.:
   - parasympatholytic drugs
   - beta-sympathomimetic drugs
   - illicit drugs
➤ Endogenous adrenaline/anxiety
	➤ Prolonged activity/stimulation
	➤ Chronic hypoxemia
	➤ Compensatory response to transient hypoxemia
	➤ Chorioamnionitis
	➤ Cardiac rhythm abnormalities
	➤ Anemia

BASELINE FHR BRADYCARDIA

When the fetal heart rate is below 110 bpm for ten minutes or more, it is called bradycardia (Figure 7.3—next page). This distinguishes a baseline change from a prolonged deceleration, which is defined as a visually apparent decrease in FHR from the baseline that is greater than or equal to 15 bpm, lasting greater than or equal to two minutes but less than ten minutes. One practical issue with this definition is that few providers wait at least ten minutes to move toward delivery given a sudden, pronounced drop in the baseline FHR, but often refer to "fetal bradycardia" as the indication for delivery. Technically, it should be called a prolonged deceleration, and the length of time it subsequently takes to deliver the infant determines whether it crosses the semantic line into bradycardia. An exception is mild bradycardia (90 to 109 bpm), which is not necessarily concerning if present with moderate variability and accelerations. In these cases, the baseline just happens to be slightly below the generally accepted range. Pathologic bradycardia usually is due to parasympathetic suppression of the sinus and atrioventricular nodes, to the point of a complete heart block. The ventricle has a pacemaker set at about 60 bpm. When FHR is normal, the pacemaker never has reason to discharge, but if there is complete or nearly complete heart block, it activates and prevents asystole. This is why fetal bradycardias rarely drop below 60 bpm. An FHR slower than this generally is a sign of serious fetal depression or cardiac dysfunction (Figure 7.4). If the FHR is less than 90 bpm in the absence of congenital heart block, the likelihood of fetal hypoxemia or hypoxia increases.

Figure 7.3: Fetal Bradycardia—FHR less than 110 bpm for Greater Than or Equal to Ten Minutes

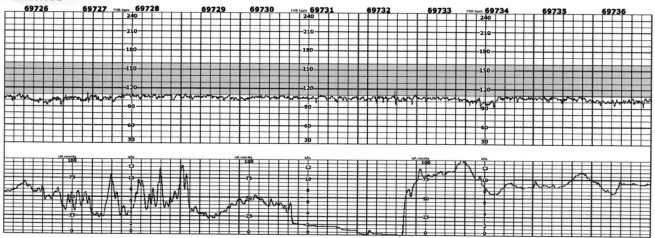

Figure 7.4: Fetal Bradycardia—Progressive from 110 to Less Than 60, Suggestive of Severe Hypoxia and Agonal FHR Tracing

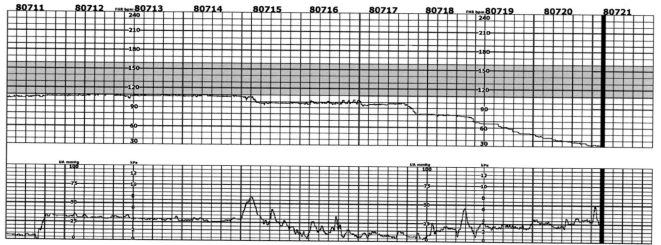

76

Table 7.2: Causes of Baseline FHR Bradycardia

Maternal	Fetal
➢ Supine positioning ➢ Hypotension ➢ Connective tissue diseases ➢ Prolonged hypoglycemia ➢ Hypothermia ➢ Medication or drug response	➢ Umbilical cord occlusion/prolapse ➢ Decompensating fetus ➢ Cardiac conduction defects ➢ Cardiac anatomic defects ➢ Maturity of the parasympathetic nervous system ➢ Excessive/prolonged parasympathetic (vagal) stimulation

Bradycardia is assessed by duration, degree of variability, and presence or absence of accelerations. The etiology may be idiopathic, fetal, maternal, or both maternal and fetal (Table 7.2).

When persistent bradycardia is observed, it is important to determine quickly whether the bradycardia is a true FHR or actually the maternal pulse (Figure 7.5). This can be confirmed by either taking the maternal pulse while listening to the monitor, or if time permits, by performing a brief ultrasound of the FHR and comparing it with the maternal heart rate. This applies to external as well as internal monitoring techniques. When there is a question of congenital heart block, ultrasound allows visualization of atrial and ventricular motion, and whether they are concordant or beating independently of one another (dissociated). In complete heart block, the atria beat at one rate, and the ventricles at an unrelated different rate.

Figure 7.5: Fetal Heart Rate Tracing Showing Maternal and Fetal Pulse at Almost the Same Baseline Rate

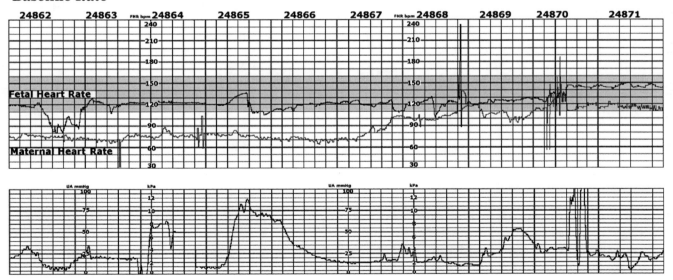

WANDERING BASELINE

At times, the baseline may be difficult to determine (Figure 7.6—next page). Extending the time of monitoring and correlating it with the clinical picture should lead to an accurate interpretation. Care should be taken to assure that the cardiotachometer is adequately recording to time any decelerations with contractions. Internal monitoring (if possible) also may be helpful to establish baseline. In some cases of progressive fetal compromise, the baseline loses variability and begins to "wander" due to deteriorating neurologic function, a finding that can portend an agonal pattern or underlying fetal brain anomaly.

Figure 7.6: Wandering Baseline

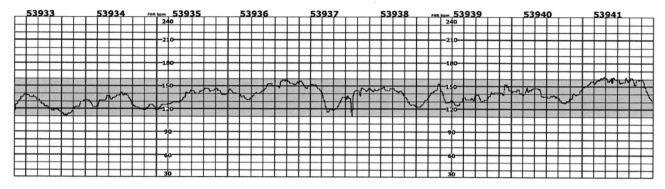

DEFINING FHR VARIABILITY

The term, **baseline FHR variability**, is used to describe moment-to-moment fluctuations in the FHR. Variability is a product of integrated activity between the more immature sympathetic and more mature parasympathetic branches of the autonomic nervous system. (See Chapter 3 for a full discussion on the functioning of the autonomic nervous system.) The sympathetic nerves stimulate increases in FHR, while the parasympathetic systems cause decreases in FHR.

Concurrent activity of the two components of the autonomic nervous system leads to numerous small increases and decreases in the FHR, giving the tracing a jagged appearance. Baseline FHR variability, therefore, reflects the status and oxygenation of the central nervous system through its effects on the heart. For variability to be normal, the basal oxygen needs of the fetus must be met. Normal variability is associated with normal (or near-normal) fetal pH.

Variability is a measure of the amplitude of rapid FHR excursions from peak to trough. It should be at least two cycles per minute and usually more. The National Institute of Child Health and Human Development (NICHD Consensus Panel, organized by the National Institutes of Health (NIH), makes no distinction between short-term variability (beat-to-beat

Figure 7.7: Cardiotachometer versus FSE.
Note the difference in variability recording with different tracing methods.

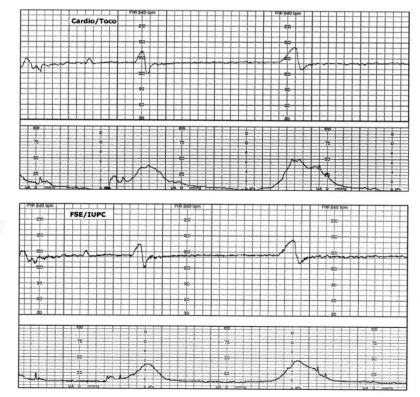

variability) and long-term variability (including accelerations and decelerations). Degree of variability is classified as:

- Absent (amplitude range is undetectable).
- Minimal (amplitude range greater than undetectable to less than or equal to 5 bpm).
- Moderate (amplitude range of 6 to 25 bpm above baseline).
- Marked (amplitude range of greater than 25 bpm above baseline).

In clinical situations, both beat-to-beat and long-term fluctuations are taken as a unit to represent overall variability.

Using contemporary fetal monitor units, external (Doppler) and internal (FSE) recordings can look similar. In Figure 7.7 (previous page), the top panel is obtained by an external cardiotachometer, while the bottom panel is recorded simultaneously using an FSE. While accelerations and decelerations are similar for both, the variability is recorded more accurately in the bottom panel.

EVALUATION OF MINIMAL FHR VARIABILITY

Absent variability has the appearance of a straight line (as if drawn with a ruler; Figure 7.8), while minimal variability appears more like a slightly shaky attempt at a line drawn without a ruler (Figure 7.9).

Figure 7.8: Absent Variability

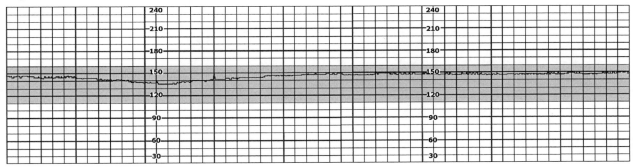

Figure 7.9: Minimal Variability

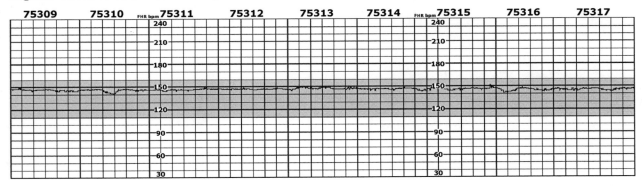

Minimal variability can have either fetal or maternal causes (Table 7.3—next page). As labor progresses and in the absence of sedating or beta-blocking medications, a tracing that had moderate variability but becomes minimal may represent an early sign of fetal acidosis, although more often simply means that the fetus is in a sleep state. The differentiation requires close observation and the presence or absence of baseline fetal heart rate changes and decelerations.

Absent variability is rare and raises concern for either moderate-to-severe acidosis or neurologic catastrophe. If variability had been present and now is absent, unless there has been use of medications known to severely suppress variability, there usually are concurrent decelerations and delivery is indicated. A possible exception is when a patient presents with a completely flat tracing with no decelerations. This is a possible presentation of fetal brain death, and if the cervix is dilated, it may be one of the few remaining occasions when fetal scalp pH can prevent an unnecessary cesarean delivery. If fetal pH can be shown to be normal, such a tracing is most consistent with preexisting devastating neurologic injury, an injury that will not benefit from an emergency cesarean section.

Table 7.3: Causes of Minimal Baseline FHR Variability

Maternal	Fetal

➤ Medication or drug response, e.g.:
  - Central nervous system depressants
  - Morphine
  - Nalbuphine hydrochloride
  - Butorphanol
  - Alcohol
  - Methadone
	➤ Sleep cycles
	➤ Central nervous system anomalies
	➤ Prolonged or severe hypoxia
	➤ Cardiac anomalies
	➤ Persistent tachycardia
	➤ Excessive/prolonged parasympathetic (vagal) stimulation

MARKED VARIABILITY

For reasons not entirely clear, early fetal hypoxemia sometimes may manifest itself as exaggerated or marked variability. Marked variability requires observation and correlation with the clinical picture and associated FHR characteristics, but it does not mandate any specific measures (or delivery) by itself.

SINUSOIDAL AND SINUSOIDAL-LIKE FHR BASELINES

Despite extensive discussion in the obstetric community, there continues to be a lack of consensus regarding the characteristics that constitute a "true" sinusoidal FHR pattern. A true sinusoidal pattern is considered a Category III FHR tracing in the 2008 NICHD nomenclature and suggests fetal acidosis and/or anemia. True sinusoidal tracings are rare, although sometimes what used to be called "long-term variability" can be confused with it.

Definition of Sinusoidal-Like FHR Baseline

The most widely accepted criteria for identifying "true" sinusoidal FHR patterns (Figure 7.10—next page) is from the NICHD Workshop Report on Electronic Fetal Heart Rate Monitoring (Macones et al., 2008): "visually apparent, smooth, sine wave-like, undulating pattern in the FHR baseline with a cycle frequency of three to five per minute that persists for greater than or equal to 20 minutes." This FHR tracing is a pattern of fixed, uniform, FHR fluctuations that create a pattern resembling successive sine waves. These oscillations do not qualify as "variability" but, instead, should be referred to as sinusoidal oscillations.

Figure 7.10: Sinusoidal FHR Secondary to Severe Fetal Anemia

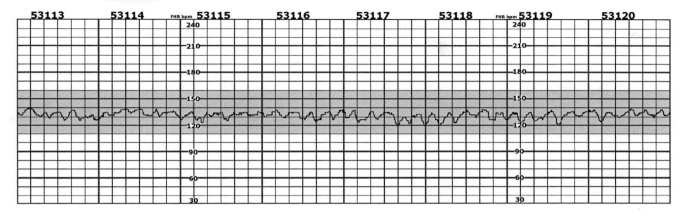

Interpretation of Sinusoidal-Like FHR Baseline

Care must be taken to distinguish these tracings from those sinusoidal-like FHR patterns that are transient and self-limited and may occur following the administration of medications. In a study by Murphy et al. that included a sample of 1,520 patients, 15% of the patients demonstrated these transient and self-limited patterns, most commonly after maternal administration of certain narcotic analgesics during labor. Because of this, not all cases of seemingly sinusoidal patterns necessitate intervention; when there is some variability or accelerations, continued observation is appropriate. Often, these sinusoidal-like (which used to be called pseudosinusoidal) tracings will revert to normal, which is not characteristic of true sinusoidal patterns. (Figure 7.11)

Figure 7.11: Sinusoidal-Like Tracing Secondary to Medication Administration
Note: This pattern resolved in less than ten minutes without intervention

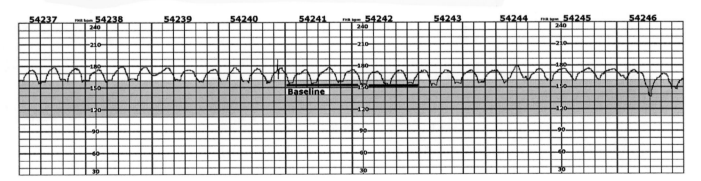

Physiology of a Sinusoidal FHR Pattern

The physiologic basis for the development of a "true" sinusoidal FHR pattern continues to be elusive. Fetal heart rate variability is known to be affected by fetal hypoxemia. Research in fetal lambs has shown that anemic fetuses exhibiting sinusoidal FHR patterns have elevated levels of arginine vasopressin, a pituitary hormone with vasopressor and antidiuretic effects. In these animal studies, administration of arginine vasopressin in the absence of cerebral ischemia, however, did not result in sinusoidal FHR patterns. The combination of elevated levels of arginine vasopressin <u>and</u> cerebral ischemia were necessary to elicit sinusoidal FHR patterns.

"True" sinusoidal FHR patterns are associated with the following fetal conditions that result in either severe fetal anemia or severe/prolonged fetal hypoxia with acidosis.

- Chronic fetal anemia associated with erythroblastosis fetalis, often from Rh sensitization
- Acute, intrapartum asphyxia
- Fetal-maternal hemorrhage
- In-utero fetal hemorrhage (e.g., ruptured vasa previa)

Interventions for a Sinusoidal FHR Pattern

When a sinusoidal FHR pattern is noted, this is a Category III FHR tracing, and immediate intervention is required. Continuous, careful fetal assessment is necessary, including ultrasound to rule out fetal hydrops, anomalies, and placental abnormalities. Ultrasound also provides an opportunity to perform a biophysical profile and quantitative fetal health parameters. When there is suspicion for fetal anemia in the very preterm fetus, percutaneous umbilical blood sampling (PUBS) under ultrasound guidance is a technique that permits fetal hemoglobin levels to be assessed and blood transfusions to be given directly to the fetus. A maternal serum Kleihauer-Betke test, which quantitates the presence of fetal blood in maternal circulation, may be helpful if a fetal-maternal hemorrhage is suspected. Preparations for a possible emergent delivery should be initiated if intrauterine resuscitation is not effective.

CONCLUSION

Baseline FHR and variability aid in assessing adequacy of fetal oxygenation. It is essential that each be interpreted in the clinical context rather than as isolated entities. In other words, the "big picture" always should be kept in mind.

RELATED READINGS

1. Association of Women's Health, Obstetric, and Neonatal Nurses (2015). <u>Fetal Heart Rate Monitoring Principles and Practices</u> (Ed. 5), Washington, D.C.: AWHONN.

2. American College of Obstetricians and Gynecologists (2009). Intrapartum fetal heart rate monitoring: Nomenclature, interpretation, and general management principles. <u>Practice Bulletin #106.</u>

3. American College of Obstetricians and Gynecologists (2010). Management of intrapartum fetal heart rate tracings. <u>ACOG Practice Bulletin #116.</u>

4. American Academy of Pediatrics and American College of Obstetricians and Gynecologists (2017). <u>Guidelines for Perinatal Care</u> (Ed. 8).

5. Freeman RK, Garite TJ, and Nageotte MP (2003). Uterine contraction monitoring (Chapter 5). IN: <u>Fetal Heart Rate Monitoring</u> (Ed. 3), Baltimore, MD: Lippincott Williams and Wilkins, pp. 54-62.

6. Freeman RK, Garite TJ, and Nageotte MP (2003). Basic pattern recognition (Chapter 6). IN: <u>Fetal Heart Rate Monitoring</u> (Ed. 3), Baltimore, MD: Lippincott Williams and Wilkins, pp. 63-89.

7. Garite TJ (2017). Intrapartum fetal evaluation (Chapter 15). IN: SG Gabbe, JR Niebyl, JL Simpson, et. al (Eds.) <u>Obstetrics: Normal and Problem Pregnancies</u> (Ed. 7), Philadelphia, PA: Churchill Livingston.

8. Macones GA, Hankins GDV, Spong CY, Hauth J, and Moore T (2008). The 2008 National Institute of Child Health and Human Development Workshop Report on Electronic Fetal Monitoring: Update on Definitions, Interpretation, and Research Guidelines. <u>American College of Obstetricians and Gynecologists.</u> 112:661-6.

9. Thorp JM (2018). Clinical aspects of normal and abnormal labor (Chapter 36). In: R Resnik, CJ Lockwood, TR Moore, et. al (Eds.) <u>Creasy and Resnik's Maternal-Fetal Medicine: Principles and Practice</u> (Ed. 8), Philadelphia, PA: Saunders Elsevier.

10. Young BK, Katz M, and Wilson SJ (1980). Sinusoidal fetal heart rate. I. Clinical significance. <u>American Journal of Obstetrics and Gynecology</u>, 136, 587-593.

Chapter 7 Review
Fetal Heart Rate Monitoring: Technology, Baseline and Variability

1.   The cardiotachometer used for external FHR monitoring produces a signal by:

   A.   measuring the time-interval difference between one R-wave of the QRS complex and the next.
   B.   detecting the strength of each contraction of the fetal heart.
   C.   transmitting a reflection of the ultrasound waves that are produced by the moving heart.

2.   True or False. In order to correctly interpret an FHR baseline, you must have at least one minute of an identifiable baseline segment in a ten-minute window.

   A.   True
   B.   False

3.   Fetal heart rate variability:

   A.   can be measured during decelerations or accelerations.
   B.   is calculated by the amplitude of the increase in FHR above the baseline.
   C.   is reflective of fetal central nervous system status.

4.   Minimal FHR variability may be attributed to:

   A.   medication or drug response.
   B.   fetal central nervous system anomalies.
   C.   fetal sleep cycles.
   D.   prolonged sympathetic stimulation.
   E.   all of the above.
   F.   A, B, and C only.
   G.   A, C, and D only.

5.   Baseline FHR bradycardia is defined as:

   A.   fetal heart rate less than 160 bpm, persisting for greater than or equal to 20 minutes.
   B.   fetal heart rate less than 110 bpm, persisting for greater than or equal to 20 minutes.
   C.   fetal heart rate less than 160 bpm, persisting for greater than or equal to 10 minutes.
   D.   fetal heart rate less than 110 bpm, persisting for greater than or equal to 10 minutes.

Chapter 7 Review Answers
Fetal Heart Rate Monitoring:
Technology, Baseline & Variability

1.   **The correct answer is C.**

2.   **The correct answer is B.** To correctly interpret a fetal heart rate baseline, you must have at least two minutes of discernible baseline over a ten-minute period.

3.   **The correct answer is C.** Fetal heart rate variability is the result of the interplay between the parasympathetic and sympathetic nervous systems. The presence of moderate variability indicates that the autonomic nervous system is functioning and well oxygenated. Variability should be evaluated between decelerations or accelerations, and it is a range of change, not an increase above baseline.

4.   **The correct answer is F.**

5.   **The correct answer is D.**

Chapter 8

Accelerations and Decelerations

INTRODUCTION

Fetal heart rate (FHR) patterns are associated with various underlying fetal conditions including responses to normal conditions, adaptive responses to transient episodes of decreased oxygenation, and impaired responses to significant hypoxia. Audible fetal heart tones first were described in the early 1800s, and slow fetal heart rates (bradycardias) were first linked to unfavorable neonatal outcomes later that century. It took another century, however, for specific FHR patterns to be related to underlying pathologic conditions. In 1946, decelerations were reported following occlusion of the umbilical cord in fetal goats, and similar decelerations were described in humans in 1959. Then, starting in the late 1950s, Hon categorized decelerations into early, variable, and late patterns. In time, certain FHR patterns (e.g., presence of accelerations) also came to be associated with underlying pathologic conditions. In time, certain FHR patterns (e.g., presence of accelerations) also came to be associated with <u>normal</u> outcomes as well.

What we really want to know during pregnancy is whether the fetus is receiving enough oxygen. Under most circumstances, we cannot assess fetal oxygen status directly because this would require cord or scalp blood sampling. The known association of certain FHR patterns with perinatal outcome led to the use of FHR monitoring as a surrogate measure of fetal oxygenation. To make optimal use of the information available through FHR monitoring and understand its nuances, however, interpretation of the FHR tracing should not consist of mere pattern recognition but also should include understanding of the physiology behind the various patterns. Fetal heart rate tracings should not be interpreted in isolation but must be correlated with physiologic changes due to gestational age, medications, and maternal medical conditions.

ACCELERATIONS

<u>Definitions of Accelerations</u>

According to the 2008 National Institute of Child Health and Human Development (NICHD) Workshop Report on Electronic Fetal Monitoring, an acceleration is a visually apparent abrupt increase in FHR of less than 30 seconds from onset to peak. A deceleration is the exact opposite, a visually apparent <u>decrease</u> and return to the FHR baseline. In fetuses of 32 weeks' gestation or greater, an acceleration is an increase in amplitude of 15 beats or greater above the baseline FHR lasting for at least 15 seconds (Figure 8.1). Before 32 weeks, an acceleration is defined as an increase of 10 beats or greater above baseline lasting for at least ten seconds. Accelerations lasting longer than two minutes, but less than ten minutes in duration, are defined as prolonged. An increase or decrease in the FHR greater than ten minutes is defined as a baseline change.

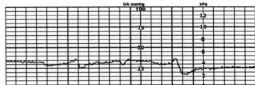

Figure 8.1: Accelerations

<u>Physiology of Accelerations</u>

Accelerations most commonly occur in the antepartum period, in early labor, and in association with variable decelerations. Most accelerations are accompanied by fetal movements, whether or not perceived by the mother. Whether the movement elicits the transient increase in FHR or whether both are a simultaneous manifestation of a common neurologic discharge is uncertain. Besides fetal movements, accelerations may occur with uterine contractions, partial compression of the umbilical cord, or with an external stimulus (e.g., scalp stimulation or vibroacoustic stimulation). Accelerations are an indicator of normal fetal oxygenation, and their presence reliably predicts both an intact autonomic nervous system and the absence of fetal metabolic acidemia at the time they are observed. The theory is that, when hypoxemic, the fetus conserves oxygen by decreasing movements such that the stimulus for accelerations also decreases. The converse is that, when normally oxygenated, movements do occur with their accompanying FHR increases.

Although accelerations are consistent with adequate oxygenation, the absence of accelerations during the intrapartum period is not necessarily alarming. Absence of accelerations may be due to normal fetal sleep cycles (which increase with gestational age) or due to medications such as narcotics and magnesium sulfate. The fetus often is inactive during labor, and other features such as degree of variability and presence of decelerations should be incorporated when determining fetal status. According to the current three-tier system for categorizing intrapartum FHR tracings, Category I tracings are normal and are strongly predictive of normal fetal acid-base status; accelerations may be present or absent in a Category I fetal heart rate tracing (see Chapter 10 for more on Categorizations of FHR Tracings).

Differentiating Accelerations

It may be difficult at times to distinguish accelerations from periodic changes in the FHR, or from a high degree of variability. Occasionally, a return to baseline following a prolonged acceleration can be mistaken for a deceleration, or the converse may occur: the rise in FHR following a deceleration may be mistaken for an acceleration (Figure 8.2). To make this distinction correctly, baseline FHR first must be established, and the relationship of the observed patterns correlated with fetal movements. If it appears that there is active fetal movement at "baseline" but that seeming-decelerations occur whenever the fetus stops moving, one most likely is seeing prolonged accelerations with "decelerative" returns to baseline. If there has been an established baseline that appeared to decline but now has increased again, this increase may be the resolution of a prolonged mild deceleration rather than an acceleration per se. In terms of distinguishing accelerations from variability, the practitioner must guard against the temptation to mistake compensatory increases in FHR following decelerations for "normal" accelerations and be falsely reassured. Examples include "shoulders" on variable decelerations, or overshoot following resolution of a prolonged deceleration.

Figure 8.2: Brief Return to Baseline Within a Deceleration

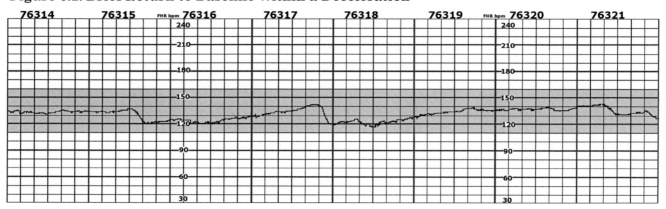

DECELERATIONS

According to the 2008 NICHD Workshop Report on Electronic Fetal Monitoring, a deceleration is a visually apparent decrease in FHR baseline. In order to fully assess decelerations and their impact on the FHR tracing, the provider must understand the different varieties of decelerations, early, variable, and late, as well as the physiology behind each. The provider also must assess if the decelerations are periodic, meaning associated with contractions, or episodic, which are changes that occur in the absence of contractions. Additionally, the provider should determine if the decelerations are recurrent or have resolved with intervention.

EARLY DECELERATIONS

Definition of Early Decelerations

An early deceleration (Figure 8.3) is a visually apparent, usually symmetric, gradual decrease and return of the FHR baseline with a nadir in greater than or equal to 30 seconds associated with a uterine contraction (Table 8.1—next page). The early deceleration occurs simultaneously with the uterine contraction in a mirror-image fashion. During a contraction, myometrial compression of the fetal head gradually increases and then gradually decreases, with the drop in FHR mirroring the timing of the contraction. Early decelerations are so-named only because they are not "late" (see below), and perhaps because "timely deceleration" did not sound quite right.

Figure 8.3: Early Decelerations

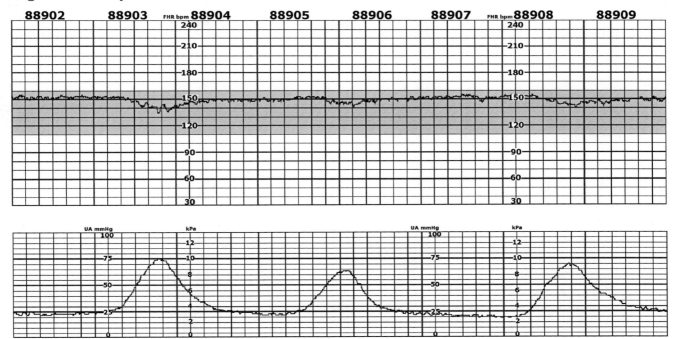

Early decelerations occur simultaneously with contractions, and the nadir (lowest point) of the decelerations coincides with the peak of the contractions, when pressure on the fetal head is the greatest. They rarely fall more than 30 to 40 bpm below the baseline FHR and, therefore, often are described as shallow decelerations. Early decelerations are uniform in appearance; i.e., they look similar to one another in shape, except that stronger contractions often result in deeper early decelerations.

Physiology of Early Decelerations

The sinoatrial (SA) node is a group of pacemaker cells in the right atrium of the heart that controls the heart rate. The SA node is influenced by the autonomic nervous system, which has two components, sympathetic and parasympathetic, components that have opposite actions on organs. For the heart, parasympathetic signals travel through the vagus nerve and cause release of the neurotransmitter, acetylcholine, at the SA node, slowing the heart rate. In contrast, sympathetic nerves traveling along blood vessels release norepinephrine, increasing the heart rate.

Table 8.1: 2008 NICHD Workshop Report Definition of Early Decelerations

> - Visually apparent, usually symmetric, *gradual* decrease and return of the FHR associated with a uterine contraction.
> - A *gradual* decrease in onset to nadir of greater than or equal to 30 seconds.
> - The decrease is calculated from the onset to the nadir of the deceleration.
> - The nadir of the deceleration occurs at the same time as the peak of the contraction.
> - In most cases, the onset, nadir, and recovery of the deceleration are coincident with the beginning, peak, and ending of the contraction, respectively.

Although the exact mechanism of early decelerations has not been proven, compression of the fetal head during contractions is believed to precipitate a reflex vagal response, slowing discharge from the SA node and decreasing FHR. Compression of the fetal head increases pressure within the skull, decreasing intracranial blood flow and increasing carotid artery downstream resistance. Given relatively constant cardiac output (CO), blood pressure (BP) is proportional to resistance (R) or (BP = R x CO); thus, when R increases, so does BP. Baroreceptors (receptors that detect changes in pressure) sense this increase in blood pressure. In an effort to normalize pressure, reflex baroreceptor-mediated parasympathetic signals slow the heart to decrease cardiac output, resulting in a deceleration that occurs in proportion to the degree of head compression. Although our understanding of the mechanism of early decelerations has not been proved, pressure applied using fingers or round pessaries over the fetal skull and anterior fontanel during labor elicit similar decelerations.

Interpretation of Early Decelerations

Early decelerations are thought to be benign and likely represent a normal response to the common stimulus of head compression. They generally are not associated with fetal hypoxia, acidosis, or adverse perinatal outcome. Perhaps the most important aspect of these decelerations is that they must be differentiated from other, more serious, types of decelerations. A satisfactory recording of contractions is essential to time decelerations; otherwise, early decelerations can be indistinguishable from late decelerations, leading to inappropriate management. Moderate baseline FHR variability may aid in distinguishing the two, because it is present in the FHR baseline between early decelerations. The shape of an early deceleration should be gradual, smooth, and shallow, distinguishing it from mild variable decelerations which tend to be asymmetric even though they also may coincide with contractions. It is important to understand that some FHR tracings will demonstrate concurrent early and variable decelerations, making this distinction even more difficult.

Factors Associated with Early Decelerations

Although it would seem that fetal head compression would occur in virtually all labors, in fact, classic early decelerations clinically are uncommon, occurring in only 5% to 10% of labors. Vertex presentation, active labor, the second stage of labor, and decreased amniotic fluid volume all increase the likelihood that the fetal head will be compressed by a contraction and increase the likelihood of early decelerations as a response. Early decelerations also are associated with primigravidity, a higher incidence of cephalopelvic disproportion (CPD), and persistent occiput posterior presentation.

Management of Early Decelerations

Management of early decelerations is simple: no intervention is required! The only critical issue is that care providers must differentiate them accurately from variable and late decelerations.

VARIABLE DECELERATIONS

Definition of Variable Deceleration

As the name implies, variable decelerations come in many shapes, sizes, and timings (Table 8.2). They can occur ante- or intrapartum and are named appropriately, for—much like snowflakes—no two are exactly alike. Even though they are common, the variety in their appearance can complicate interpretation.

"Classic" variable decelerations consist of a small acceleration (the primary acceleration) followed by an abrupt drop in the fetal heart rate with onset to nadir occurring over less than 30 seconds (Figure 8.4). The classic variable deceleration then resolves as abruptly as it begins and finishes with a small acceleration (the secondary acceleration or "shoulder").

Table 8.2: 2008 NICHD Workshop Report Definition of Variable Decelerations

> ➤ Visually apparent, *abrupt* decrease in FHR, defined as less than 30 seconds from the onset of the deceleration to the beginning of the nadir.
>
> ➤ The decrease in FHR is calculated from the onset to the nadir of the deceleration.
>
> ➤ The decrease in FHR is greater than or equal to 15 beats per minute, lasting greater than or equal to 15 seconds, but less than or equal to two minutes in duration.
>
> ➤ When associated with uterine contractions, their onset, depth, and duration commonly vary with successive uterine contractions.

Figure 8.4: Variable Decelerations

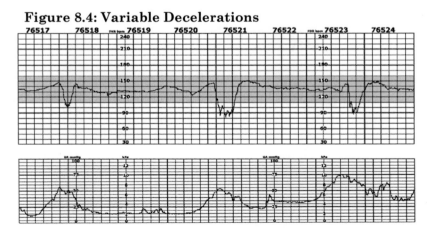

93

The pattern during the deceleration portion often has a spiked, jagged, V-shaped appearance (or occasionally are U- or W-shaped), sometimes with accelerative components. Variability is present during the deceleration. The depth of the deceleration can vary from 15 beats to greater than 60 beats below baseline, and the duration can range from 15 seconds to two minutes. Timing in relation to a contraction is, characteristically, variable: many variable decelerations occur during contractions, but variable decelerations can occur between contractions, or in the absence of contractions.

Characteristics of Variable Decelerations

In a sense, variable decelerations can be viewed as a normal physiologic response to a transient stress and, thus, indicate that the fetal autonomic nervous system is intact. Variable decelerations are consistent with normal fetal oxygenation if they resolve completely with normal FHR features between one such deceleration and the next. (Table 8.3)

Table 8.3: Components of Variable Decelerations that Suggest Fetal Well-Being

> ➤ FHR decelerations generally last no longer than 40 to 60 seconds on a repetitive basis.
>
> ➤ Return of FHR to baseline is abrupt. There are no persistent "late components" manifested by a slow return or a late deceleration with the return.
>
> ➤ Baseline FHR is not increasing.
>
> ➤ FHR variability is not decreasing.

Adapted from Freeman-Garite (2003)

Physiology of Variable Decelerations

Variable decelerations result from decreased fetal perfusion due to compression of the umbilical cord. When mechanical compression occurs, the thin-walled, low-pressure vein becomes occluded first. Blood no longer can return from the placenta to the fetal circulation but still can exit the fetus via the unimpeded umbilical arteries. The decreased venous return to the heart precipitates a sympathetic nervous system response, resulting in a transient, reflex tachycardia that is seen as the initial, anterior shoulder in the classic variable deceleration. If the pressure on the umbilical cord continues and becomes greater, the small, thicker-walled, higher-pressure umbilical arteries also are compressed. The placenta is a low-resistance shunt within the fetal circulation, and compressing the umbilical arteries effectively stops flow through it, removing the shunt and leaving fetal blood to flow through the remaining, higher-resistance, fetal systemic circulation. The net effect is a sudden increase in systemic vascular resistance (SVR), which increases BP and activates the parasympathetic nervous system through the fetal baroreceptors. Reflex vagal stimulation occurs, abruptly decreasing the FHR. Once compression of the umbilical cord begins to lessen, the higher-pressure arteries open first, while the umbilical vein remains compressed, resulting in lowering of SVR and BP, cessation of vagal stimulation, and an increase in FHR. If there again is a brief period of decreased venous return to the heart, the sympathetic system is reactivated and a transient tachycardia (posterior shoulder) may occur. As perfusion in the umbilical vein resumes, the BP normalizes, the parasympathetic and sympathetic systems come into balance, and the FHR returns to baseline.

Interpretation of Variable Decelerations

Variable decelerations are the most common decelerations observed during labor. Some of the factors associated with variable decelerations are listed in Table 8.4 (next page). Clearly, most of these factors can lead to increased umbilical cord compression or decreased ability of the umbilical cord to tolerate compression.

Transiently reduced umbilical cord perfusion generally is well tolerated by healthy fetuses. If reduced umbilical cord perfusion is persistent and prolonged enough, however, fetal PO_2 falls and carbon dioxide (CO_2) accumulates such that fetal PCO_2 rises and a respiratory acidosis occurs. If umbilical cord occlusion is prolonged for five to ten minutes, oxygen deprivation can lead to the cells shifting to inefficient anaerobic metabolism, generating organic acids and a metabolic acidosis as buffers are consumed (see Chapter 4 on Fetal Oxygen and Acid-Base Metabolism).

Even if umbilical cord compression is not prolonged, repetitive, frequent occlusions may not give the fetus time to compensate between episodes, such that there is a gradual decline in PO_2, a rise in PCO_2, and a deterioration of pH. The most important measure of fetal status during these episodes is from the baseline heart rate characteristics noted *between* variable decelerations. Again, normal baseline, variability, and accelerations imply normal oxygenation between episodes of umbilical cord compression. Gradual loss of these intervening features may portend fetal decompensation.

Several attempts have been made to classify the severity of variable decelerations on the basis on depth and duration. The clinical utility of these classifications has been questioned. Certain aspects of variable decelerations may correlate with impaired fetal oxygenation, however. Krebs et al. (1983) examined the frequency and

Table 8.4: Factors Associated with Variable Decelerations

> Velamentous insertion of the umbilical cord

> Battledore placenta (eccentric cord insertion)

> Short umbilical cord

> Nuchal cord

> Umbilical cord malposition or body entanglement

> Occult or obvious prolapsed cord

> Rapid descent of the fetus

> Decreased amniotic fluid volume

> Knot in the umbilical cord

> Decreased Wharton's jelly—the gelatinous layers of cord that help to cushion the umbilical cord and prevent compression.

significance of various features of variable decelerations and identified characteristics associated with a higher incidence of fetal hypoxemia. These factors are the opposite of those listed in Table 8.3 (previous page) including decelerations lasting longer than 40 to 60 seconds, slow return to baseline, increasing baseline FHR, and decreasing baseline FHR variability. When any of these factors are present during a variable deceleration, further evaluation and possible intervention is warranted.

Management of Variable Decelerations

When variable decelerations are noted, the attendant first should note their frequency, appearance, resolution characteristics, and baseline between decelerations. Next, it is important to consider the clinical context (antepartum versus intrapartum, membrane status, presence of fetal growth restriction or oligohydramnios, stage of labor, etc.). Intrapartum, variable decelerations in a tracing otherwise retaining variability, accelerations, and normal baseline do not require intervention; these can be observed. Variable decelerations that are noted antepartum during a nonstress test often warrant ultrasonographic assessment to rule out oligohydramnios, which can increase the risk of umbilical cord compression. It must be added that, because variable decelerations are so common in FHR tracings, most of these are not associated with oligohydramnios; the reflex ultrasound obtained after variable decelerations are noted during nonstress testing usually shows normal amniotic fluid volume. Finally, the provider must assess if the decelerations are periodic, meaning associated with contractions, or episodic, which are changes that occur in the absence of contractions.

Recurrent Variable Decelerations

Recurrent variable decelerations are those occurring with more than 50% of the uterine contractions. Recurrent variable decelerations or those that occur in conjunction with other FHR abnormalities are associated with lower fetal cord pH and hypoxia. In an attempt to relieve umbilical cord and vena caval compression, the pregnant woman should be repositioned onto her left or right side. If minimal or absent variability also is present, oxygen should be administered by nonrebreather mask in order to increase oxygen delivery to the fetus. If the patient is in labor, a cervical examination should be performed to rule out cord prolapse as well as to evaluate progress of labor. Intravenous fluids will increase maternal intravascular volume and may improve uteroplacental perfusion but, otherwise, will not alleviate cord compression. Amnioinfusion may be considered, especially in the setting of oligohydramnios, and may help to relieve cord compression.

Persistent variable decelerations in the latent or early-active phase of labor may, over the hours, lead to fetal hypoxemia, hypoxia, and acidosis before delivery occurs. Loss of variability and reactivity, altered baseline, or the appearance of late or prolonged decelerations may mandate interventions to hasten delivery. However, recurrent, variable decelerations may be tolerated during the second stage of labor if delivery is expected soon, and if FHR baseline variability is maintained. Five-minute Apgar scores usually are normal following such a delivery, although the one-minute score may be low. This low one-minute Apgar score is due to a respiratory acidosis that resolves as soon as the newborn breathes off the carbon dioxide that was retained during the episodes of cord compression. An infant with a low one-minute Apgar score who responds well to resuscitation is not a cause for concern.

LATE DECELERATIONS

Definition of Late Decelerations

Late decelerations (Figure 8.5—next page) are shallow, uniformly shaped decelerations that are characterized by a gradual decrease from and subsequent return to baseline. The 2008 NICHD Workshop Report (Table 8.5) defines late decelerations as a "visually apparent, usually symmetric, *gradual* decrease and return of the FHR associated with a uterine contraction." A "gradual" decrease is further defined as the elapse of time from the onset of the deceleration to its nadir being greater than or equal to 30 seconds. The nadir of the deceleration must occur <u>after</u> the peak of the contraction, although the extent to which they are offset is not strictly defined.

Table 8.5: 2008 NICHD Workshop Report Definition of Late Decelerations

> ➤ Visually apparent, usually symmetric, gradual decrease and return of the FHR associated with a uterine contraction.
>
> ➤ A gradual FHR decrease is defined as from the onset to the FHR nadir of greater than or equal to 30 seconds.
>
> ➤ The decrease in FHR is calculated from the onset to the nadir of the deceleration.
>
> ➤ The deceleration is delayed in timing, with the nadir of the deceleration occurring after the peak of the contraction.
>
> ➤ In most cases, the onset, nadir, and recovery of the deceleration occur after the beginning, peak, and ending of the contraction, respectively.

Figure 8.5: Late Decelerations

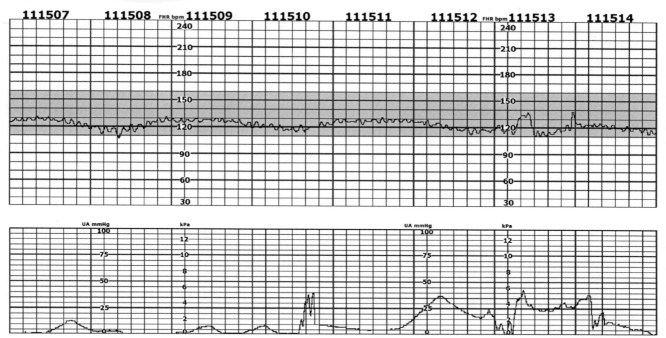

Likewise, there is no minimum required degree of deceleration and clinically, the magnitude of the deceleration does not correlate well with fetal outcomes. In fact, as is addressed later, sometimes the most subtle late decelerations can be the most concerning. Despite these relatively straightforward definitions, intra- and inter-observer agreement about the presence or absence of late decelerations can be suboptimal, and disagreement sometimes will exist even among experienced practitioners.

Physiology of Late Decelerations

Uterine contractions compress the maternal spiral arterioles that traverse the myometrium, temporarily decreasing placental perfusion (Figure 8.6). During the contraction, with less maternal blood flow in the intervillous spaces, less oxygen is transferred into the fetal circulation. As a result, fetal PO$_2$ declines. The normal placenta has considerable reserve and still can transfer adequate amounts of oxygen even when perfusion is reduced briefly, such that most fetuses tolerate transient reductions in PO$_2$ without an apparent physiologic response. If the placental function is compromised such that basal fetal oxygen requirements are being met— but just barely—then an additional decrease in perfusion and oxygen transfer

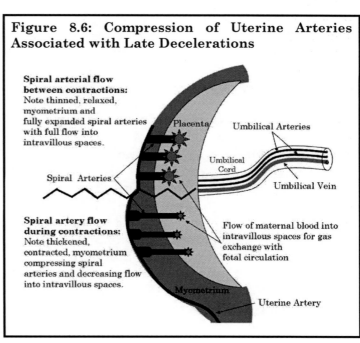

Figure 8.6: Compression of Uterine Arteries Associated with Late Decelerations

Spiral arterial flow between contractions: Note thinned, relaxed, myometrium and fully expanded spiral arteries with full flow into intravillous spaces.

Spiral Arteries

Spiral artery flow during contractions: Note thickened, contracted, myometrium compressing spiral arteries and decreasing flow into intravillous spaces.

Placenta

Umbilical Arteries

Umbilical Cord

Umbilical Vein

Flow of maternal blood into intravillous spaces for gas exchange with fetal circulation

Myometrium

Uterine Artery

97

may lower fetal PO_2 enough to elicit a physiologic fetal response. This response can occur by one (or both) of two mechanisms. First is the "classic" neurogenic late deceleration and second is direct myocardial depression due to severe hypoxia and acidosis.

Both mechanisms share some common characteristics. In the fetus with a compromised placenta, the contraction-mediated reduction in perfusion lowers the rate of oxygen transfer to the fetus. Fetal PO_2 does not fall immediately, however, because the fetus has to consume what oxygen already is in its system before its blood oxygen concentration declines, there is a lag time of up to 30 seconds. This lag time accounts for the delay in onset of a late deceleration until after the contraction is well established. Likewise, when uteroplacental oxygen transfer becomes optimal again, fetal PO_2 does not immediately rise to normal; it takes some seconds before fetal PO_2—and the physiologic response in reaction to the brief hypoxemic episode—normalizes, accounting for the delay in FHR return to baseline until after the contraction is over. These "lag times" are what account for the appearance of late decelerations.

Vagal Mechanisms

In the first (and most common) pathway believed to be associated with late decelerations, vagal and/or elevated blood pressure responses to a decrease in fetal blood oxygen concentrations are the primary mechanism. When fetal PO_2 falls below a minimal normal threshold, chemoreceptors located in the fetal aorta and carotid arteries detect this decreased PO_2 and activate the parasympathetic nervous system via the vagus nerve. The vagus nerve is a cranial nerve that innervates the sinoatrial and atrioventricular nodes, the pacemakers that control heart rate. Vagal stimulation to these pacemakers slows the heart rate. In addition to vagal nerve stimulation, changes in fetal blood pressure play a role in this mechanistic pathway. During a uterine contraction when less oxygen is available in the intervillous space, the fetus may respond by releasing norepinephrine and epinephrine. These catecholamines, in turn, produce a rise in the fetal blood pressure which, in turn, leads to a reflex bradycardia to bring blood pressure back toward normal.

Late Decelerations Due to Fetal Acidosis

In the second pathway believed to be associated with late decelerations, metabolic acidosis directly impairs the fetal myocardium. In this circumstance, a different type of late deceleration occurs when a fetus already has sustained hypoxia significant enough to shift to anaerobic metabolism and lactic acid production, leading to acidemia and eventually tissue acidosis. Severe acidosis depresses the fetal myocardium directly and may result in late decelerations that begin even closer to the onset of contractions (Figure 8.7). Also, the acidosis may depress the fetal heart so significantly that it becomes barely able to respond to further changes in parasympathetic signals. These shallow, late decelerations may be subtle

Figure 8.7: Late Decelerations Associated with Severe Acidosis
Note the subtle late decelerations on the FHR tracing after contractions. These could be easily missed.

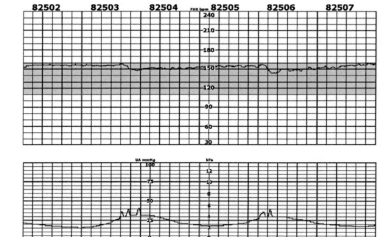

98

and possibly reflect a blunted compensatory response to significant fetal hypoxia and metabolic acidosis, and almost always are accompanied by absent variability and lack of accelerations. Often the baseline "wanders" and may portend an agonal pattern to follow if urgent delivery is not affected. Although the depth of late decelerations can vary with the intensity of contractions, the depth is not indicative of the degree of fetal hypoxia in these late decelerations in which acidosis is so severe that fetal adaptive mechanisms are lost.

Implications of Late Decelerations

While late decelerations are associated with an increased risk of hypoxia and acidosis at the time of delivery, many fetuses with late decelerations during labor essentially are healthy and ultimately have a normal (or at least acceptable) umbilical artery pH. Although late decelerations are concerning, they sometimes can be a normal response to an unusual stress (e.g., a prolonged deceleration), and vagally mediated late decelerations do not necessarily signify the presence of acidemia or acidosis *per se*. Periods of hypoxia during contractions, while preferably avoided, do not necessarily result in fetal or neonatal harm if they are not associated also with metabolic acidosis. Differentiating which fetuses with late decelerations are acidotic is not always possible before delivery, and is dependent upon the evaluation of other aspects of the FHR tracing, particularly baseline variability. Likewise, although their presence is associated with hypoxia, the presence of late decelerations is a poor predictor of hypoxic-ischemic encephalopathy when evaluated independently of the heart rate baseline or variability.

Reversible Late Decelerations

Transient events may occur that produce a single or even a brief pattern of late decelerations (e.g., maternal hypotension from an epidural anesthetic or supine positioning). These patterns are more amenable to treatment and resolution than the late deceleration associated with severe hypoxia and acidosis. There are a wide variety of precipitating factors that are associated with development of reversible late decelerations, including maternal hypotension for whatever reason, maternal hypo- or hyperventilation, hypovolemia, and uterine tachysystole. If late decelerations occur within these contexts, and resolve with therapeutic measures, then labor generally can be allowed to proceed.

The presence of recurrent late decelerations necessitates a prompt evaluation, including a search for potential underlying causes. For example, placental abruption, nonremediable umbilical cord compression, or fetal sepsis due to chorioamnionitis often requires urgent delivery. Likewise, sustained maternal acidosis of any cause generally will lead to fetal acidosis; however, the fetal acidosis may correct as the maternal condition improves without having to deliver the fetus.3

Evaluation of Late Decelerations

Late decelerations that occur sporadically are not likely to be of clinical significance. Of potentially greater concern are recurrent late decelerations. When late decelerations occur with greater than or equal to 50% of contractions, they are deemed "recurrent." The subsequent discussion of clinical management is in reference to recurrent late decelerations only.

Within the three-tier NICHD fetal heart rate interpretation system, the presence of late decelerations indicates that the tracing is not Category I; however, without an assessment of variability one cannot determine whether it is Category II or III. Unless there is a sinusoidal pattern, a Category III tracing requires absent baseline FHR variability. Late decelerations occurring in the context of minimal or moderate baseline variability only constitute a Category II tracing. This differentiation makes sense in context of the known physiologic mechanisms of late decelerations, i.e., those that occur in the setting of appropriate variability probably represent the vagal pathway described above, while late decelerations with absent variability are more likely to reflect acidosis (and acidemia), which can minimize FHR variability, leading to late decelerations through direct myocardial suppression. Thus, the fetus with absent FHR variability and late decelerations is at high risk of acidosis, while late decelerations occurring in the setting of normal variability may reflect only periods of hypoxemia during contractions which, in themselves, do not pose a threat to fetal health.

Ultimately, the management will depend upon into which tier in the NICHD schema the FHR tracing is determined to fall. Efforts should be made to resolve Category III tracings in an expedited manner. This may include the provision of supplemental oxygen, position changes, and the discontinuation of uterine stimulating agents. If the FHR tracing fails to improve with these conservative measures, then further tests of fetal well-being or expedited delivery (including potentially instrumental or cesarean delivery), depending upon the exact clinical scenario, should be considered. If the tracing is Category II, then the optimal management approach is less clear. Consideration can be given to simple conservative measures, such as position changes or supplemental oxygen; however, depending upon the exact clinical context, an expedited delivery may or may not be indicated. The NICHD recommendations for a Category II tracing are open-ended, stating that they "require evaluation and continued surveillance and reevaluation, taking into account the entire associated clinical circumstances."

Given the well-documented existence of inter-observer variability in FHR evaluations, sometimes even very experienced practitioners will disagree on whether or not late decelerations are present in a tracing. In the event that a consensus cannot be reached in this regard, it is most important for the practitioners to agree on the presence or absence of appropriate variability. If the variability is normal, then the tracing is not Category III, regardless of the presence of late decelerations. However, if the variability is minimal, even very subtle late decelerations are of significant concern, in which case it would be wise to err on the side of caution and expedite delivery.

PROLONGED DECELERATIONS

When there is a visually apparent decrease in FHR from the baseline that is greater than or equal to 15 bpm lasting greater than or equal to two minutes but less than ten minutes, it is called a prolonged deceleration. These are not synonymous with fetal compromise, but prompt evaluation is needed to rule out the various possible etiologies. Vaginal examination should be performed to check for umbilical cord prolapse and to assess the progress of labor. Additionally, one needs to be certain that it actually is the FHR that is being measured, and not the maternal pulse. This can be confirmed by performing a brief ultrasound of the FHR and comparing it with the maternal pulse. This applies to external as well as internal monitoring techniques. If internal monitoring is possible, this may be helpful to assess the fetal heart further. Oxygen, positional changes, and fluids all should be done expeditiously.

Most prolonged decelerations will resolve and labor can continue. If the deceleration has not resolved within four or five minutes despite therapeutic efforts, there should be consideration of urgent delivery, either vaginally (with or without vacuum or forceps depending upon how soon it is estimated that the patient could deliver by pushing alone) or moving to the operating room. If the patient is transferred to the operating room, a final FHR check sometimes reveals resolution of the deceleration, in which case a decision is made about whether to allow labor to continue or proceed to cesarean delivery. The latter decision depends on many factors: other FHR features, frequency of such decelerations, maternal co-morbidities, underlying pregnancy complications, and availability of operating room personnel.

CONCLUSION

Whereas FHR accelerations are considered normal and indicative of adequate fetal oxygenation, FHR decelerations are a fetal compensatory response to changes in uteroplacental perfusion, fetal blood pressure, and the intrauterine environment from many causes, most of them correctable. If decelerations are present, a careful assessment of potential etiologies should be performed and the appropriate series of therapeutic maneuvers applied. Additionally, the provider must assess if the decelerations are periodic, meaning associated with contractions, or episodic, which are changes that occur in the absence of contractions. Confronted with recurrent decelerations, particularly when there are other characteristics of the tracing that are concerning, decisions about the route of delivery depend on the estimated time to delivery. The decisions should take into account the presence or absence of associated abnormalities in the FHR baseline and variability, as well as stage and rate of labor progression and any maternal conditions that may be present. The entire maternal-fetal unit must be viewed as a whole to assure the best possible outcomes for both mother and baby.

RELATED READINGS

1. American College of Obstetricians and Gynecologists (2010). Management of intrapartum fetal heart rate tracings. <u>ACOG Practice Bulletin #116</u>.

2. Chauhan SP, Klauser CK, Woodring TC, Sanderson M, Magann EF, and Morrison JC. (2008). Intrapartum nonreassuring fetal heart rate tracing and prediction of adverse outcomes: interobserver variability. <u>American Journal of Obstetrics and Gynecology</u>, 199: 623.e1-5.

3. Freeman RK, Garite TJ, and Nageotte MP (2003). Basic pattern recognition (Chapter 6). IN: <u>Fetal Heart Rate Monitoring</u> (Ed. 3), Baltimore, MD: Lippincott Williams and Wilkins, pp. 63-87.

4. Freeman RK, Garite TJ, and Nageotte MP (2003). Physiologic basis of fetal monitoring (Chapter 2). IN: <u>Fetal Heart Rate Monitoring</u> (Ed. 3), Baltimore, MD: Lippincott Williams and Wilkins, pp. 8-21.

5. Garite TJ (2007). Intrapartum fetal evaluation (Chapter 15). IN: SG Gabbe, JR Niebyl, and JL Simpson (Eds.) <u>Obstetrics: Normal and Problem Pregnancies</u> (Ed. 5), Philadelphia, PA: Churchill Livingston, pp. 365-392.

6. Hofmeyr GJ (2008). Amnioinfusion for potential or suspected umbilical cord compression in labor. <u>The Cochrane Library.</u> Issue 4, 1-38.

7. Larma JD, Silva AM, Holcroft CJ, Thompson RE, Donohue PK, and Graham EM. (2007). Intrapartum electronic fetal heart rate monitoring and the identification of metabolic acidosis and hypoxic-ischemic encephalopathy. <u>American Journal of Obstetrics and Gynecology</u>, 197:301, e1-8.

8. Macones GA, Hankins GDV, Spong CY, Hauth J, and Moore T (2008). The 2008 National Institute of Child Health and Human Development workshop report on electronic fetal monitoring: Update on definitions, interpretation, and research guidelines. <u>American College of Obstetricians and Gynecologists</u>, 112:661-6.

Chapter 8 Review
Accelerations and Decelerations

1. The type of FHR deceleration that results from decreased intracranial pressure and increased blood pressure due to increased carotid artery downstream resistance is a(n):

   A. early deceleration.
   B. late deceleration.
   C. variable deceleration.

2. The anterior shoulder of a "classic" variable deceleration is the result of the _____ _____ being compressed and stimulation of the _____ nervous system.

   A. umbilical artery, parasympathetic
   B. umbilical artery, sympathetic
   C. umbilical vein, parasympathetic
   D. umbilical vein, sympathetic

3. If umbilical cord compression is prolonged five to ten minutes, the decrease in PO_2 will result in a metabolism shift to _____ and a _____ acidosis.

   A. aerobic, respiratory
   B. aerobic, mixed
   C. anaerobic, metabolic
   D. anaerobic, respiratory

4. The primary mechanism thought to be associated with late decelerations is the vagal response due to a decrease in fetal blood oxygen concentrations. This vagal response occurs as a result of stimulation from the:

   A. baroreceptors.
   B. chemoreceptors.
   C. both A and B.
   D. neither A nor B.

5. Select the correct statement regarding the presence or absence of accelerations in an FHR tracing.

   A. The presence of FHR accelerations reliably predicts the absence of fetal metabolic acidemia.
   B. The absence of FHR accelerations reliably predicts acidemia.
   C. Both A and B are correct.
   D. Neither A nor B are correct.

Chapter 8 Review Answers
Accelerations and Decelerations

1. **The correct answer is A.** Early decelerations are the result of head compression that results in increased intracranial pressure, decreasing intracranial blood flow, and increasing carotid artery downstream resistance, resulting in an increase in blood pressure. This is sensed by the baroreceptors that activate the parasympathetic nervous system.

2. **The correct answer is D.**

3. **The correct answer is C.** When cells are deprived of oxygen for a long period of time, in order to maintain the body's survival, they will shift their metabolism to anaerobic, and metabolic acidosis will be present.

4. **The correct answer is C.** Chemoreceptors measure oxygen saturation and carbon dioxide levels. Baroreceptors measure pressure changes—blood pressure, intravascular volume, and cardiac output. Both are responsible for late decelerations via activating the parasympathetic system.

5. **The correct answer is A.**

Chapter 9

Antepartum Fetal Assessment

INTRODUCTION

The purpose of fetal heart rate (FHR) monitoring is to assess whether the fetus is adequately oxygenated. Ultrasound adds the ability to assess fetal anatomy, amniotic fluid volume, growth, blood flow, and the quantitation of biophysical variables. If the obstetric provider is knowledgeable about the different aspects of fetal monitoring and the physiology behind them, he or she is more likely to respond appropriately to abnormal patterns. This chapter will discuss the tests used to assess the fetus during the antepartum period, including nonstress testing (NST), vibroacoustic stimulation (VAS), biophysical profile (BPP), and contraction stress testing (CST).

NONSTRESS TESTS

The NST is the most widely used technique for monitoring fetal oxygenation status (often referred to by the general and imprecise term "fetal well-being"). Nonstress testing is common not because it is the best testing modality, but because it is noninvasive, easy to do, and serves as a quick screening measure to determine whether further testing and assessment is necessary. Fetal heart rate accelerations (described in Chapter 7) are the standard measure of the test. Accelerations correlate with normoxia and, when paired with oscillations and fluctuations of the FHR around the baseline (variability), imply an intact autonomic nervous system. The concept is that an adequately oxygenated fetus will have a functional autonomic nervous system that will send sympathetic and parasympathetic signals to the heart, and that an adequately oxygenated heart will respond to these signals with certain normal patterns (normal baseline rate, moderate variability, and occasional accelerations). In this sense, FHR patterns are surrogate measures of fetal oxygen status. Because all fetal oxygen derives from the placenta, the NST indirectly is testing adequacy of placental function, too. NSTs generally are performed in pregnancies in which there is increased risk of fetal hypoxemia or death due to either maternal or fetal factors (Table 9.1). For conditions in which the fetus is at risk from factors not related to lack of oxygen (e.g., most structural fetal anomalies), nonstress testing is not indicated because it is designed only to assess one factor—lack of oxygen. For example, a fetus with bilateral renal agenesis that is 100% lethal after delivery may have a normal antepartum NST; but certainly, this fetus is not doing well.

Table 9.1: Common NST Indications

> - Chronic renal disease
> - Collagen vascular disease
> - Decreased fetal movement
> - Diabetes mellitus
> - Hypertensive disorders
> - Fetal growth restriction
> - Isoimmunization
> - Multiple gestation
> - Post-term pregnancy
> - Previous unexplained fetal demise
> - Oligohydramnios

Performing Nonstress Tests

The NST is performed while the patient reclines in the semi-Fowler's position. External monitors are placed on the maternal abdomen. The FHR is monitored by a Doppler ultrasound cardiotachometer, and a tocodynamometer is used to monitor uterine contractions. An event marker is given to the patient to indicate each time that the fetus is felt moving. Women should not fast prior to the NST, and those that have continued to smoke despite recommendations should not smoke for several hours before the NST as both of these factors may affect the NST. The blood pressure is recorded before the start of the NST and repeated if outside the normal range. The tracing usually lasts 20 minutes but can be extended up to 40 minutes if necessary. Occasionally, one records normal FHR patterns in just a few minutes when the fetus is very active. It may be acceptable to end the test sooner than 20 minutes in such cases; however, the tracing generally is continued for the full 20 minutes to check for decelerations or other changes in heart rate.

Nonstress Test Interpretation

An NST is classified as either being reactive or nonreactive. For most patients, a reactive NST is considered normal and correlates well with fetal survival over the next week. Reactivity is determined by the presence of FHR accelerations and is defined as two accelerations of either 15 beats (or ten beats for fetuses less than 32 weeks) above the baseline, lasting at least 15 seconds from beginning to end (or ten seconds if less than 32 weeks), within a 20-minute segment of the FHR tracing (Figure 9.1, Table 9.2). Computerized FHR interpretation has the benefit of objectively interpreting the findings, which translates into potentially better positive and negative predictive accuracy and fewer equivocal tests at gestational ages earlier than 32 weeks. It does not incorporate clinical context, however; the same borderline-reactive tracing that is deemed reactive in a woman with a marginal indication for nonstress testing may be interpreted by human assessment quite differently in the hypertensive, diabetic woman with lupus and growth-restricted twins. Other parameters noted in the NST include baseline fetal heart rate, variability, and the presence or absence of fetal heart decelerations. The significance of a reactive NST with decelerations is unclear. Variable decelerations frequently are recorded during an NST, especially at earlier gestational ages. These decelerations generally are benign, but ultrasound to rule out oligohydramnios, or prolonged FHR monitoring, may be required depending on the depth and duration of the deceleration(s).

Table 9.2: Interpretation of NST

> - Reactivity is determined by presence of two accelerations in a 20-minute period.
>   - For fetuses greater than or equal to 32 weeks, accelerations must be 15 beats above the FHR baseline and of 15 seconds duration.
>   - For fetuses less than 32 weeks, accelerations must be ten beats above the FHR baseline and of ten seconds duration.

Figure 9.1: NST Tracing

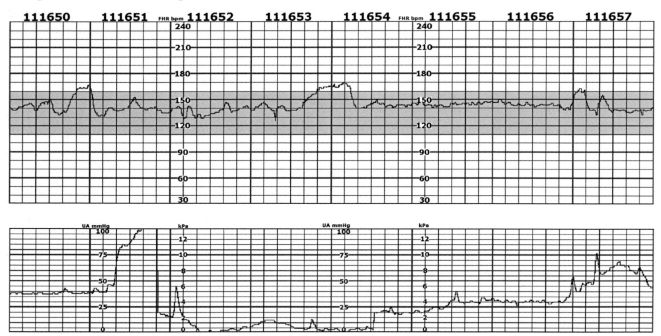

Timing of Nonstress Testing

Nonstress testing can be done at any gestational age at which the fetus is viable for delivery. This means NSTs can be done as early as 23 to 24 weeks but usually are begun at or after 32 weeks because of the potential need for delivery. Doing NSTs before viability does not make sense, because if there were an ominous pattern such that stillbirth is thought likely, previable delivery, by definition, will increase the likelihood to 100%. The difficulty is that preterm fetuses do not manifest the same FHR patterns as do term fetuses (fewer 15-beat accelerations, but more ten-beat accelerations and variable decelerations). When judged by the "term" (15-beats-for-15-seconds) criteria, many preterm NSTs will appear nonreactive (up to 75% at 24 weeks), leading to follow-up testing (usually a biophysical profile). Some providers bypass this dilemma by calling tracings in extremely preterm fetuses "strips" instead of NSTs, suggesting that a care provider will accept FHR patterns in these fetuses that do not display the features considered indicative of normal oxygenation on a "true" NST. If a 20-minute tracing is being done for fetal indications, it needs an accepted criterion for interpretation. In the case of preterm nonstress testing, when the accelerations are at least ten beats above baseline and last at least ten seconds, two such accelerations in 20 minutes are associated with similar perinatal outcomes as are two 15-beat accelerations when gestational age is 32 or more weeks. Preterm fetuses not meeting the ten-beat criterion need further assessment before nonreactivity can be ascribed to prematurity.

In general, most NSTs are begun at or after 32 weeks. The decision to initiate surveillance at early gestational ages should in part be dictated by the expected survival of the neonate, limitations of the neonatal intensive care unit, the availability of additional testing (e.g., a biophysical profile), and the ability of the physician to appropriately interpret the fetal heart rate tracing.

Because fetal behavior and sleep cycles at term may not produce accelerations in twenty minutes (10% to 12% of third-trimester fetuses), the NST may be prolonged up to 40 minutes. Almost all NSTs obtained from healthy fetuses are reactive by 40 minutes (less than 6% of third-trimester fetuses will have a nonreactive NST). Those fetuses, mostly likely, will undergo further testing by biophysical profile. It may not always be feasible to continue the NST for longer than 20 minutes, however, and further testing such as a biophysical profile can be performed to assess fetal status further. A biophysical profile score of 8/10 (0 points for the nonreactive NST) still is considered indicative of a normal fetal oxygenation status.

Nonstress Tests' Predictive Value

A reactive NST correlates well with fetal survival over the next week (perinatal mortality 4 to 5/1,000), and usually is repeated weekly. A nonreactive NST is associated with a perinatal mortality rate of 30 to 40/1,000; however, the false positive rate is high—between 75% and 90%. This means that a nonreactive NST must be followed up by a more comprehensive test such as a biophysical profile (see biophysical profile section). Although NSTs have a low false negative rate (i.e., appearing normal when in fact the fetus is at risk), this risk is not zero. Approximately 50% of perinatal deaths occurring within a week of a reactive NST occur from non-predictable causes (e.g., abruption, cord accident, etc.), but false positive NSTs are more frequent in certain conditions (e.g., asymmetric fetal growth restriction, diabetes mellitus, oligohydramnios, severe preeclampsia, or isoimmunization). In these cases, testing either should be more frequent (ranging from twice-weekly to daily), or additional testing methods may be indicated.

VIBROACOUSTIC STIMULATION

Vibroacoustic stimulation (VAS), also referred to as fetal acoustic stimulation (FAS), has become a common adjunct tool in the assessment of the fetus during an NST. The use of VAS reduces the number of nonreactive NSTs by 38% and shortens the time needed to gain a reactive NST by almost ten minutes. These benefits are thought to be a result of altering fetal behavior from a quiet sleep state to an active sleep state. It is not clear whether it is the sound or vibration that is stimulating the fetus.

Fetal Response to Vibroacoustic Stimulation

Studies have shown that the use of VAS increases gross fetal body movements, fetal heart rate variability, and the frequency and duration of accelerations. The fetal vibratory sense is developed fully between 22 to 24 weeks and the ability to hear begins to develop about a month later. Fetal response to VAS is believed to be brought about by activating the auditory pathways in the central nervous system. When the central nervous system is activated, fetal accelerations as well as an increase in fetal heart rate variability occur. The auditory system is thought to be one of the first systems affected in the presence of hypoxia.

The literature suggests that most fetuses will respond to vibroacoustic stimulus from 26 weeks' gestation, though lack of response before 28 to 30 weeks' gestation may be related to the functional immaturity of the auditory pathways. Fetuses in quiet sleep with minimal heart rate variability frequently convert to moderate variability seen in active sleep when they are exposed to VAS. Researchers also theorize that transmission of vibration and sound may be impaired during labor and following rupture of membranes. Some healthy fetuses have been observed not to respond to sound stimulation during these periods.

Performing Vibroacoustic Stimulation

To perform VAS, an artificial larynx is placed onto the patient's abdomen, ideally over the fetal head. Presentation may need to be confirmed before placement. The healthcare provider should inform the patient of the indication and risk prior to utilizing vibroacoustic stimulation. Offering a demonstration of the device by applying it to a fleshy part of the patient's arm or leg may reduce anxiety or concerns about its use. The fetal heart rate baseline should be determined before the stimulus is applied to better assess fetal response.

There are no evidence-based standards for performing VAS. If the NST is nonreactive after several minutes, a VAS stimulus is applied; the time and duration of stimulus should be recorded at each application. Typically, stimulus is applied for one to five seconds. If there is no fetal response within 60 seconds, the stimulus can be repeated up to three times. The absence of acceleration after two applications of VAS is considered a negative response. Occasionally, tachycardia or bradycardia can be observed following VAS. Both of these patterns typically resolve without the need for additional intervention. However, the false-negative rate of VAS has been reported to be as high as 67%. Consequently, VAS should be performed only when there is the capability to perform a biophysical profile. Healthcare providers performing VAS should be aware of their institutions' policies regarding frequency and length of application of stimulus.

Vibroacoustic stimulation recently has been shown to decrease the number of low biophysical profile scores and increase the specificity, positive predictive value, and accuracy of NST testing.

Intrapartum VAS also has been used when there is a prolonged period without FHR accelerations, especially when there are concurrent decelerations and concern for fetal acidosis. Whereas accelerations following VAS are consistent with a non-acidotic fetus, it must be noted that a lack of response is not necessarily indicative of a fetus in jeopardy.

Concerns Regarding Vibroacoustic Stimulation

There has been concern as to whether VAS may alter fetal sleep state or cause fetal hearing loss. How much sound does the device produce? Recorded sound levels *in utero* have been measured at 60 to 85 dB and in open air at 100 to 110 dB. Studies have shown no difference in neonatal hearing acuity between those who were exposed near term to VAS and those who were not exposed. The auditory effects in fetuses who are preterm or whose health may be complicated by maternal hypertension or maternal cocaine use are not as clear. There also have been reports of prolonged decelerations following VAS, presumably from sudden fetal movements compressing the umbilical cord. Although there is potential for this to happen, one might make the case that it is better that it happens when the patient is on the monitor under medical care rather than a random time following a loud noise or sudden fetal movement for some other reason.

Summary of Vibroacoustic Stimulation

The use of VAS has been shown to reduce the incidence of nonreactive NSTs, thus decreasing time, money, and resources spent on further fetal evaluation.

BIOPHYSICAL PROFILE

The fetal biophysical profile (BPP) is a non-invasive, sonographic assessment developed to provide information about fetal health in addition to the commonly used NST. As discussed above, the NST is used widely as a screening assessment of fetal acidemia. As such, a reactive NST has proved to be a valuable measure of a healthy fetus. Unfortunately, a nonreactive NST is a poor predictor of a compromised fetus. Real-time ultrasonography allows visualization of the fetus in its environment while simultaneously permitting observation of fetal activities. These observations offer information on fetal status and provide guidance for clinical decision-making.

The components of the biophysical profile are regulated by the central nervous system (CNS) and, therefore, reflect current CNS function. Normal biophysical activity is a reliable confirmation of an intact CNS and normally oxygenated fetus. Therefore, the request for a BPP often is due to a nonreactive NST. By assessing multiple biophysical variables, the care provider may be able to differentiate between NSTs that are nonreactive for reasons other than fetal hypoxemia (false-positive) versus those truly representing fetal compromise.

Biophysical Profile Components

There are four discreet sonographic parameters of the BPP: fetal movement, fetal tone, breathing movements, and amniotic fluid measurement. The final component of the BPP, which cannot be assessed by ultrasound, is the NST result. Each of the five total components is interpreted as either present or absent, with a score of two (present) or zero (absent) assigned, respectively, for a maximum possible score of 10 (Table 9.3—next page). An odd numbered score is not possible; there is no "partial credit." A BPP test is time-limited, and must be completed in 30 minutes or less, but on average, it can be done in eight to ten minutes.

Table 9.3: Biophysical Profile Scoring Technique

Biophysical Variable	Normal (score=2)	Abnormal (score=0)
Fetal breathing movements	Greater than or equal to one episode of greater than or equal to 30 sec in 30 min	Absent or no episode of greater than or equal to 30 sec in 30 min
Fetal movement	Greater than or equal to three <u>discrete</u> body/limb movements in 30 min	Less than three episodes of body/limb movements in 30 min
Fetal tone	Greater than or equal to one episode of active extension with return to flexion of fetal limb(s), trunk, or hands	Either slow extension with return to partial flexion, or absent fetal movement
Reactive fetal heart rate	Two accelerations in a 20-minute period For fetuses greater than or equal to 32 weeks' gestation, greater than or equal to 15 bpm and of greater than or equal to 15 seconds duration For fetuses less than 32 weeks' gestation, greater than or equal to 10 bpm and of greater than or equal to ten seconds duration	Insufficient accelerations, absent accelerations in a 20-minute tracing.
Qualitative amniotic fluid volume	Single deepest vertical pocket greater than 2 cm	Either no pockets, or largest pocket less than 2 cm in vertical axis

Physiology of Biophysical Profile

Biophysical variables appear in sequence as the fetus matures. Fetal tone is the first of the parameters to function, at approximately eight weeks' gestation. Next, fetal movement occurs by nine weeks, fetal breathing movements by 20 to 24 weeks, and, lastly, fetal heart rate regulation develops. As the fetus matures, the fetal brain goes through significant organizational changes. By about 24 weeks, the fetus exhibits two patterns of fetal electrocortical function. In a variant of rapid-eye-movement (REM) sleep, the fetus during active sleep experiences episodic breathing, sporadic movement, and increased FHR variability. During non-REM or quiet sleep, in contrast, the fetus does not exhibit breathing movements and FHR variability is reduced. These two behavioral states have a diurnal rhythm, with REM dominating late evening and being least frequent in the early morning hours. The fetus oscillates between REM and non-REM sleep states every 30 to 60 minutes (in some cases, even longer). During REM sleep, oxidative metabolism of the fetal cortex increases about 25% and blood flow increases to select regions of the brain. Fetal breathing movements usually are seen during REM sleep and are episodic. The frequency of breathing increases as gestational age advances and is seen 10% to 20% of the time in fetuses between 24 to 28 weeks and 30% of the time after 30 weeks. Similarly, gross body movements are increased in REM sleep. They occur about 10% of the time after 30 weeks of gestation. These fluctuations in fetal sleep cycle and accompanying presence of BPP components should be kept in mind when evaluating fetal well-being.

Amniotic fluid volume, the primary source of which is fetal urine after the second trimester, when determined to be low by ultrasound, is an indicator of chronic adverse fetal condition. It has been suggested that during chronic impairment of fetal oxygenation, preferential shunting of blood may occur to the more vital fetal organs such as brain, heart, and adrenals. This adaptation of blood flow happens at the expense of kidney perfusion. Stress leads to secretion of pituitary vasopressin, which has an antidiuretic hormone effect on the kidney, decreasing urine output. The first four components of the BPP relate more to an acute hypoxic event, while amniotic fluid reflects chronic changes. Nevertheless, in response to a chronic decrease in oxygen availability, the fetus adjusts its behavior to conserve oxygen. Decreases in fine and gross movements reduce oxygen use by muscles. Decreased fetal breathing also reduces diaphragm (another muscle) activity. A shift from an alternating pattern of active sleep and quiet sleep to quiet sleep alone decreases oxygen consumption by the brain. Each of these changes conserves oxygen. Each can be identified by the BPP.

Indications for Biophysical Profile Testing

Women at higher-than-average risk of fetal asphyxia or intrauterine fetal demise are candidates for fetal surveillance. Some of these high-risk conditions include, but are not limited to, diabetes mellitus, chronic hypertension, fetal growth restriction, amniotic fluid abnormalities, post-term pregnancy, and various fetal anomalies. Depending on the condition, testing usually is initiated between 32 to 34 weeks, or earlier if indicated. There are no specific guidelines as to how frequently to monitor the fetus, but testing should be done at least weekly.

Complete Biophysical Profile

When performing a complete biophysical profile, all five components are assessed, and scored in a specific manner (Table 9.3—previous page). Gross body movements or rolls should occur at least three times in 30 minutes. Tone is assessed by the active opening and closing of the hand or active flexion and extension of a limb. Breathing movements should be observed for at least 30 continuous seconds. Important to this observation is that the chest wall moves in as the abdominal wall moves out, so this motion should not be confused with other gross body movements. Maternal breathing sometimes can create an illusion of fetal chest wall movement. If a question of validity exists, it is reasonable to ask the patient to hold her breath for several seconds to confirm fetal breathing. Fetal heart reactivity is determined by the same criteria as an NST; that is, two accelerations of 15 bpm above baseline and lasting 15 seconds in a 20-minute period for fetuses greater than or equal to 32 weeks' gestation.

While the above BPP parameters serve to evaluate more acute fetal status, the final measurement, amniotic fluid, is a marker of longer-term fetal oxygenation. In order to meet the criteria for "adequate," the pocket of amniotic fluid has to measure greater than or equal to 2 cm. Of note, this does not exclude oligohydramnios, because some fetuses still can meet criteria for "adequate" fluid on a BPP but have low fluid as an overall index for the gestational age. Prior to measuring, using Doppler to assure that cord and fetal parts are excluded from the pocket can be helpful.

Modified Biophysical Profile

For this version of a BPP, only an NST in conjunction with amniotic fluid volume is used. Because NST is a marker of normal acute state fetal oxygenation, and amniotic fluid of the chronic state, these two together serve as an assessment of both acute and chronic fetal condition. This is the basis for the "modified biophysical profile," which uses only NST and amniotic fluid volume. According to studies by Nageotte et al. and Miller et al., amniotic fluid volume and NST together (a modified BPP) correlate highly with normal outcome, to the same degree as the full ten-point assessment. According to Miller et al., the rate of intrauterine fetal demise within one week of a normal test is the same as for a full BPP (0.8 per 1,000 women).

Table 9.4: Interpretation of BPP Results and Recommended Clinical Management

Test Score Result	Risk Asphyxia	Perinatal Morbidity Within One Week Without Intervention	Management	% Fetal Acidemia	Corrected Mortality per 1,000
10 of 10, 8 of 10 (normal fluid), 8 of 8 (NST not done)	Risk of fetal asphyxia extremely rare	1 per 1,000	Intervention only for obstetric and maternal factors, not fetal.	13	1
8 of 10 (low fluid)	Possible chronic fetal compromise	89 per 1,000	If fetal kidneys present and intact membranes, deliver for fetal indications; if preterm, consider continued surveillance.	No data	No data
6 of 10 (normal fluid)	Equivocal test, possible fetal asphyxia	Variable	Deliver if mature; in the immature fetus, repeat within 24 hr; if persistent—deliver.	24	10
6 out of 10 (low fluid)	Probable fetal asphyxia	89 per 1,000	Deliver for fetal indications.	No data	No data
4 of 10	High probability for fetal asphyxia	91 per 1,000	Consider CST if immature; deliver if mature.	58	26
2 of 10	Fetal asphyxia almost certain	125 per 1,000	Deliver if greater than or equal to 32 weeks.	67	94
0 of 10	Fetal asphyxia certain	600 per 1,000	Deliver if greater than or equal to 32 weeks.	100	285

Adapted from: Manning FA, Platt LD, and Sipos L (1980). Antepartum fetal evaluation: Development of a fetal biophysical profile score. American Journal of Obstetrics and Gynecology, 136:787. Manning FA (2011). Chapter 23 Fetal Biophysical Profile Score: Theoretical Considerations and Practical Application IN: Sonography in Obstetrics and Gynecology (Ed. 7), Fleischer, Toy, Lee, Manning, Romero (Ed.), McGraw-Hill Professional.

Interpretation of the Biophysical Profile

The loss of each component of the BPP is sequential, and each serves as a different marker of fetal condition. Therefore, decreased reactivity and breathing motions best correlate with early hypoxemia, while loss of body movement and tone imply longer duration or greater severity of impaired oxygenation. Accordingly, if reactivity of the NST and normal amniotic fluid are present, then neither acute nor chronic hypoxemia is likely. Overall, the rate of intrauterine fetal demise within one week secondary to placental causes after a normal BPP (8 or 10/10) is low (0.8 per 1,000 women).

Management Based on the Biophysical Profile Score

Management decisions based on BPP scores must take into consideration each individual component of the evaluation and not focus on total score alone. Both Manning (1991) and

Vintzileos (1987) have offered management plans for combinations of BPP results as well as multiple others (Table 9.4—previous page).

Summary of the Biophysical Profile

For all of its utility, the BPP is not perfect. It allows a graded prognosis of fetal morbidity and mortality, but until the score reaches zero, there still will be some neonates without morbidity (Figure 9.2). Certain medications (magnesium sulfate, narcotics, beta-adrenergic blockers, etc.) may decrease the BPP score independent of oxygen status, and some fetal anomalies may interfere with movement or fetal urine production (and, thus, amniotic fluid), artificially lowering the score. Amniotic fluid may be low after rupture of membranes, regardless of fetal oxygenation. For these reasons, low BPP scores may be misleading under these circumstances. At term, the chance of an adverse outcome by delivering based on a falsely low BPP is small, but in severely preterm fetuses, delivery may lead to significant morbidity or death from sequelae of prematurity. In these cases, the clinician must be convinced that the risk of continuing the pregnancy outweighs the risk of delivery.

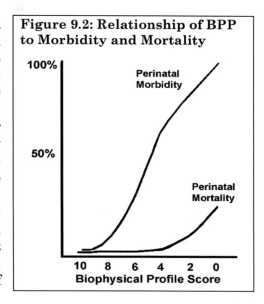

Figure 9.2: Relationship of BPP to Morbidity and Mortality

Advantages of BPP scoring are clear in clinical settings. Because multiple variables are assessed, the score is graded, rather than "all or none." A normal score has excellent predictive value for good outcome (fetal anomalies notwithstanding). It combines both acute and chronic measures and allows for detection of changes in fetal condition. One single testing method cannot provide all of the information needed for clinical decision-making. The BPP comes closest of any current antepartum test to providing an accurate, least-invasive assessment of fetal health.

CONTRACTION STRESS TESTS

Placental Physiology

The placenta normally operates with considerable reserve, at up to 150% of what is required to meet basal fetal oxygen delivery requirements. The price for operating at maximal capacity is that the placenta cannot further increase its oxygen delivery capacity if the fetus becomes hypoxemic. The benefit, however, is that this reserve allows the placenta to continue to meet fetal requirements under many adverse conditions such as minor abruptions, small infarcts, or in any circumstances in which uterine artery perfusion is decreased. While not every pregnancy is complicated by these conditions, most pregnancies are complicated by intermittent uterine artery compression—and subsequently decreased placental perfusion—that occurs every two to three minutes for the hours that constitute labor. If the placenta were not able to compensate for these regular periods of decreased perfusion and oxygen delivery, fetal hypoxia and acidosis would be the rule of every labor.

In some pregnancies, however, the placenta functions with less reserve, sometimes at or just above what is required minimally to support the fetus, or even below that level. This is called uteroplacental insufficiency. This condition puts the fetus at risk, and depending on gestational age and the risks of prematurity, the risk of continued pregnancy may outweigh the risk of delivery. Of the several available antenatal tests to assess fetal status, the contraction stress test (CST) specifically evaluates uteroplacental function. Whereas NST is non-provocative and does nothing to stress the maternal-fetal system, a CST involves inducing contractions and observing the FHR response to these episodes of decreased placental perfusion and lower oxygen transfer, essentially measuring the degree of placental reserve. With normal placental reserve, the fall in fetal PO_2 during a contraction is not enough to elicit a fetal cardiovascular response, and the FHR pattern appears normal. When reserve is marginal, however, the fall in fetal PO_2 during a contraction may "cross the threshold" into physiologic hypoxemia, manifested as late decelerations in the FHR tracing that may have appeared reactive before the stress of contractions. When reserve already is below the minimum threshold, the FHR often is nonreactive even before the appearance of late decelerations during the CST.

Utility of Contraction Stress Testing

Most of the time, a reactive NST is adequate assessment of baseline fetal oxygen status. The most common reason for CST use is following a nonreactive NST, equivocal BPP, and/or uncertainty of further clinical management. In situations where no obvious signs of fetal compromise exist and yet fetal well-being cannot be confirmed based on above test results, CST may be a useful additional tool. It can help differentiate between nonreactivity due to impaired placental function from a false positive result.

In recent decades, BPP testing largely has taken the place of CSTs, because the BPP is non-invasive, has no contraindications, and gives information about amniotic fluid and fetal anatomy. In the occasional patient, however, a CST still can be helpful (e.g., severe prematurity, fetal central nervous system anomalies, or maternal medications that cross the placenta and affect the fetal nervous system, all of which can lower the BPP score even when oxygenation is normal).

Technique for Contraction Stress Testing

A CST may be spontaneous or obtained by two methods: nipple stimulation or intravenous oxytocin infusion (oxytocin challenge test, or OCT). A nipple stimulation CST is reasonably safe, simple, and effective, and it offers the advantage of being non-invasive. The patient is placed in a semi-Fowler's or left lateral tilt position to prevent supine hypotension. An initial 20 to 30 minutes of monitoring is performed to establish baseline FHR and presence of accelerations or decelerations. If three contractions occur spontaneously in a ten-minute period with an appropriately reactive FHR response and no late decelerations, the test is considered negative and complete. If no contractions occur, the patient stimulates her own nipples (or a partner may assist). Generally, she is instructed to pull and roll one nipple between her thumb and forefinger gently, usually through her clothing. She continues to do this until she perceives uterine tightening or for a maximum of two minutes, then stops. Alternatively, a breast pump can also be used. If a frequency of three contractions in ten minutes is not achieved, then an additional two minutes of nipple stimulation is implemented after five minutes of rest. This method has been shown to be as safe and effective as oxytocin-induced CSTs, and may be completed in half the time, on average 40 minutes, including the preceding 20-minute tracing.

If nipple stimulation is ineffective or if the woman does not feel comfortable with it, the CST becomes an OCT through the use of oxytocin. An intravenous line is started and dilute solution of oxytocin is infused. Depending on the protocols of the institution, the rate of oxytocin is increased every 30 to 40 minutes until three contractions lasting 40 to 60 seconds occur in ten minutes. There is no requirement as to how intense the contractions have to be. When the three-contractions-in-ten-minutes threshold has been reached, oxytocin is discontinued and the patient is observed on the monitor until her contractions have subsided. Although the CST usually is safe, possible complications are uterine tachysystole, uterine tetany leading to fetal bradycardia, or stimulation of actual labor.

Interpretation of Contraction Stress Tests

Contraction stress test results are interpreted the same regardless of the technique used, categorized into one of the five following categories:

Negative (80% to 90%): (suggestive of a non-hypoxic fetus) depending on the population being tested. There are no late FHR decelerations or significant variable FHR decelerations with a contraction frequency of at least three in a ten-minute period (Figure 9.3). A negative result indicates adequate placental function and has been associated with a perinatal loss rate of less than 1/1,000 pregnancies over the following week.

Figure 9.3: Negative CST

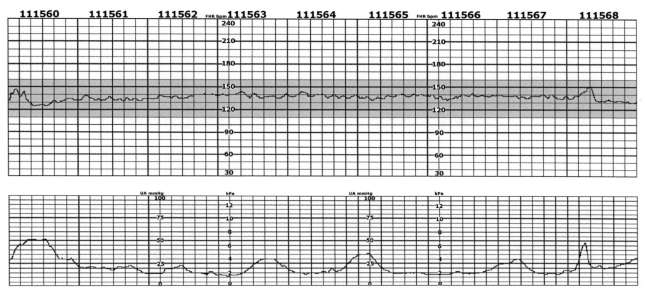

Positive (5%) (suggestive of placental insufficiency): A CST is interpreted as positive when there are late FHR decelerations following 50% or more of contractions, even if the contraction frequency is less than three contractions in ten minutes (Figure 9.4—next page). This is most concerning when associated with decreased variability, absence of FHR accelerations, or decreased fetal movement. A positive result is consistent with some degree of uteroplacental insufficiency. Intervention should be considered, but management depends on gestational age and maternal risk factors. Positive predictive values for perinatal mortality or morbidity after a positive CST range from 9% to 70%, depending on the population, the outcome assessed, and whether the NST that was completed prior to the CST was reactive or nonreactive. A nonreactive NST followed by a positive CST (nonreactive-positive) is associated with a much worse outcome (risk of stillbirth 88/1,000) than a reactive NST followed by a positive CST (reactive-positive) (risk of stillbirth less than 1/1,000). The likely reason is that the reactive-positive indicates a fetus that is receiving adequate basal oxygen before the additional stress of contractions, whereas the nonreactive-positive indicates a fetus already is hypoxemic even before the CST was started. The "false-positive" rate of a positive CST is between 30% and 91% (varying with the definition of adverse outcome) and most fetuses with a positive test tolerate labor. For this reason, a positive result should be interpreted with caution and management based on gestational age and the rest of the clinical scenario.

Figure 9.4: Positive CST

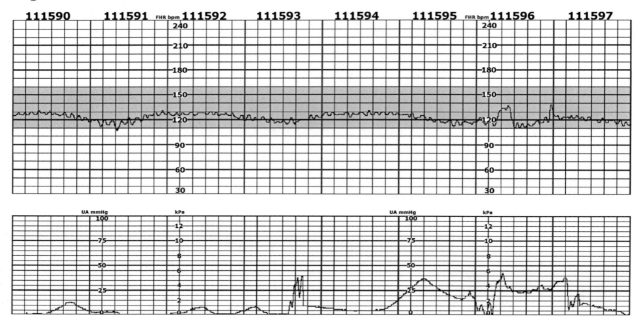

Equivocal or Suspicious (10%) (suggestive of placental insufficiency): A CST is interpreted as suspicious when there are intermittent late FHR decelerations or significant variable FHR decelerations. This result occurs infrequently. Generally, a suspicious CST is repeated in 24 hours, or is considered in conjunction with an amniotic fluid volume (AFV) or BPP. The risk of fetal demise does not appear to be increased for those patients who repeat testing within a day of a suspicious CST.

Unsatisfactory: Poor quality recording, particularly in the late phase of the contraction or frequency of uterine contractions less than three per ten minutes. Repeat testing usually will be more successful. If repeating a CST is not feasible, then testing with BPP is appropriate.

If tachysystole occurs during the test and there are no late decelerations, the test is interpreted as negative. However, if FHR decelerations occur in the presence of uterine tachysystole, retesting with avoidance of tachysystole should be carried out before the test can be interpreted as satisfactory. Late decelerations during tachysystole may be a normal fetal response to an exaggerated stress rather than a sign of uteroplacental insufficiency.

Contraindications to Contraction Stress Tests

Because a CST involves contractions and the small chance of inducing labor, it cannot be done in cases in which labor is contraindicated. There is reasonable evidence, however, that a CST does not increase the rate of preterm delivery if used appropriately. Relative contraindications to the CST generally include conditions associated with possible preterm labor, uterine rupture, or uterine bleeding (Table 9.5).

Table 9.5: Contraindications to CST

> Prior classic cesarean section (vertical uterine scar)
> Preterm labor
> Cervical insufficiency with cerclage
> Placenta previa or suspected abruptio placentae
> Polyhydramnios*
> Multiple gestation*
> Preterm premature rupture of membranes*

*Relative contraindication

Summary of Contraction Stress Tests

Although healthcare providers may be able to detect a fetus that is at high risk with the CST, there are limitations with this form of assessment. The invasive nature of the CST, certain contraindications, and "false positives" have limited its use and led most clinicians to use BPP testing in the place of CSTs. Today, CSTs are most helpful when a BPP is unavailable or borderline, when possible delivery of a severely preterm fetus is being contemplated based on an unexpectedly low BPP score, or when a CST from spontaneous contractions occurs during a nonreactive NST. The CST occasionally helps dictate route of delivery: a fetus with a negative CST is likely to tolerate labor, whereas labor is less likely to be tolerated in the setting of a positive CST, especially if associated with a nonreactive NST. As always, clinical judgment in the management of a high-risk pregnancy is important.

CONCLUSION

The purpose of antenatal assessment is to assess fetal oxygenation. The healthcare provider needs to be aware of the physiology underlying this testing so that the best test for the patient's clinical situation can be chosen. Unfortunately, none of the testing options are perfect, so the provider must be able to correlate the patient's situation and the fetal physiology to the interpretation of the results and interventions. This allows the provider to react appropriately to the fetal antepartum testing.

RELATED READINGS

1. American College of Obstetricians and Gynecologists (1999). Antepartum fetal surveillance. <u>ACOG Technical Bulletin #9</u>. Washington D.C.

2. American College of Obstetricians and Gynecologists (2010). Management of intrapartum fetal heart rate tracings. <u>ACOG Practice Bulletin #116</u>. Washington D.C.

3. American College of Obstetricians and Gynecologists (1994). Diabetes and pregnancy. <u>ACOG Technical Bulletin #200</u>.

4. Cunningham FG, Gant NF, Leveno KJ, Gilstrap LC, Hauth JC, and Wenstrom KD (2001). Antepartum assessment (Chapter 40). Endocrine disorders (Chapter 50). <u>Williams Obstetrics</u> (Ed. 21). New York, NY: The McGraw-Hill Companies, Inc., pp. 1095-1110.

5. Druzin ML, Smith JF, Gabbe SG, and Reed KL (2007). Antepartum fetal evaluation (Chapter 11). Antepartum fetal evaluation (Chapter 12). IN: SN Gabbe, JR Niebyl, and JL Simpson (Eds.) <u>Obstetrics: Normal and Problem Pregnancies</u> (Ed. 4), Philadelphia, PA: Churchill Livingston, pp. 267-300.

6. East CE, Smith R, Leader LR, Henshall NE, Colditz PB, Tan KH (2005). Vibroacoustic stimulation for fetal assessment in labour in the presence of a nonreassuring fetal heart rate trace. <u>Cochrane Database Systematic Reviews, 18(2)</u>:CD004664.

7. Freeman RK, Garite TJ, and Nageotte MP (2003). Antepartum fetal monitoring (Chapter 12). Clinical management of nonreassuring fetal heart rate patterns (Chapter 9). IN: <u>Fetal Heart Rate Monitoring</u> (Ed. 3), Baltimore, MD: Lippincott Williams & Wilkins, pp. 181-202.

8. Grivell RM, Alfirevic Z, Gyte GM, Devane D (2010). Antenatal cardiotocography for fetal assessment. <u>Cochrane Database Systematic Reviews</u>, 20(1):CD007863.

9. Harman CR (2004). Assessment of fetal health (Chapter 21). IN: RK Creasy, R Resnik, JD Iams, CJ Lockwood, and TR Moore (Eds.) <u>Creasy and Resnik's Maternal-Fetal Medicine: Principles and Practice</u> (Ed. 6), Philadelphia, PA: W.B. Saunders.

10. Heymann MA, Rudolph AM. (1974). Cardiovascular responses to hypoxemia and acidemia in fetal lambs. <u>American Journal of Obstetrics and Gynecology</u>, 120(6):817.

11. Huddleston JF (2002). Continued utility of the contraction stress test? A critique of fetal surveillance tests. <u>Clinical Obstetrics and Gynecology</u>, 45(4):1005-1014.

12. Kaur S, Picconi JL, Chadha R, Kruger M, and Mari G (2008). Biophysical profile in the treatment of intrauterine growth-restricted fetuses who weigh <1000 g. <u>American Journal of Obstetrics and Gynecology</u>, 199:264.e1.

13. Landon MB, Catalano PM, and Gabbe SG (2001). Diabetes mellitus (Chapter 32). IN: SG Gabbe, JR Niebyl, and JL Simpson (Eds.) <u>Obstetrics: Normal and Problem Pregnancies</u> (Ed. 4), Philadelphia, PA: Churchill Livingston, pp. 1081-1116.

14. Association of Women's Health, Obstetric, and Neonatal Nurses (2009). <u>Fetal Heart Rate Monitoring Principles and Practices</u> (Ed. 4), Washington, D.C.: AWHONN.

Chapter 9 Review

Antepartum Fetal Assessment

1. True or False. A nonstress test (NST) is a fetal surveillance test based on the premise that a fetus with an intact, well-oxygenated central nervous system will accelerate its heart rate in response to fetal movement.

   A. True
   B. False

2. True or False. Recurrent variable decelerations that are seen in the antepartum period during an NST should be evaluated by ultrasound for evaluation of amniotic fluid volume.

   A. True
   B. False

3. Vibroacoustic stimulation:

   A. is indicated for 38% of patients having an NST.
   B. is best utilized during labor.
   C. should be used routinely to shorten the time necessary to complete an NST.
   D. reduces the incidence of nonreactive NSTs.

4. When evaluating the results of a biophysical profile (BPP), which of the following is true?

   A. A fetus at 26 weeks' gestation is expected to demonstrate breathing movements 30% of the time.
   B. Low amniotic fluid volume reflects chronic changes rather than an acute event.
   C. A BPP of 6 out of 10 indicates probable fetal asphyxia and immediate delivery is recommended.

5. Contraction stress tests are:

   A. a fetal assessment method to help determine placental oxygen reserve during contractions.
   B. interpreted as negative if there are no late or variable decelerations with a contraction frequency of at least three contractions in a ten-minute period.
   C. most often performed following a nonreactive NST and an equivocal BPP.
   D. all of the above.

Chapter 9 Review Answers
Antepartum Fetal Assessment

1. **The correct answer is A.**

2. **The correct answer is A.** Variable FHR decelerations can be indicative of umbilical cord compression. One instance when umbilical cord compression may occur is when there is low amniotic fluid volume.

3. **The correct answer is D.**

4. **The correct answer is B.** After the second trimester, fetal urine is the major contributor to amniotic fluid. When chronic impairment of fetal oxygenation occurs, blood is shunted to the more vital organs—heart, brain, and adrenal glands. Renal perfusion diminishes, decreasing urine output.

5. **The correct answer is D.**

Chapter 10

Fetal Heart Rate Monitoring Interpretation

INTRODUCTION

Electronic fetal monitoring (EFM) is a technique that enables healthcare providers to assess the fetal heart rate (FHR) and uterine activity continuously. The FHR is controlled by the autonomic nervous system. The autonomic nervous system consists of a balance between the well-developed parasympathetic division working to decrease the FHR and the less mature sympathetic division working to increase the FHR. The FHR varies depending on which of these divisions is more strongly "pushing" the system.

The parasympathetic and sympathetic divisions receive their input from baroreceptors (stretch receptors) that detect changes in blood pressure, and chemoreceptors that detect changes in the intrinsic factors of fetal O_2 and CO_2 levels and acid-base balance. It should be remembered that the intrinsic environment of the fetus is dependent on the extrinsic factors of the mother. Maternal factors such as maternal uptake of oxygen, uteroplacental flow, and the condition of the placenta, therefore, often influence the intrinsic factors and cause changes in FHR.

SYSTEMATIC EVALUATION OF ELECTRONIC FETAL MONITORING

When evaluating electronic fetal monitoring, the provider needs to take a stepwise approach to evaluation so that they develop an understanding of the entire maternal-fetal unit (Table 10.1). The contraction tracing should first be assessed to determine if it is internal intrauterine pressure catheter (IUPC) or external tocodynamometer. The contraction pattern should be established, and if an internal monitor is used, the strength of the contractions and the baseline uterine tone also should be noted. Attention then should be turned to the fetal heart rate (FHR). Again, the provider should determine if this is internal fetal scalp electrode (FSE) or external cardiotachometer. The FHR baseline should then be established, outside of any periodic or episodic change. The variability of the baseline should then be determined. Any accelerations and/or decelerations should be noted. As the uterine contraction pattern already has been established, the provider also can assess if any noted decelerations are periodic (associated with contractions) or episodic (occurring in the absence of contractions). The provider then can assign a category to the tracing, and begin interpretation of the EFM within the entire clinical context of the mother and fetus.

Table 10.1: Systematic Evaluation of EFM

1. Contraction pattern, including baseline and strength (if internal monitoring)
2. Baseline
3. Variability
4. Accelerations
5. Decelerations, including determination of periodic or episodic change
6. Category of FHR tracing
7. Interpretation of the FHR tracing within the current clinical context

UTILITY OF FHR TRACINGS

The FHR patterns are used to assess fetal oxygenation and reflect the complex physiologic relationship between mother and fetus. Evaluation of the FHR tracing is meant to allow the healthcare provider to determine when the fetal acid-base balance is normal or abnormal, and when to intervene to prevent adverse neonatal outcome. Although EFM is known to have a limited ability to predict cerebral palsy, its use, compared to no EFM during labor, has been shown to decrease the incidence of neonatal seizures. Presumably, this is because EFM may allow intervention before hypoxia results in fetal neurologic injury. Electronic fetal monitoring also has been associated with an increase in the rate of operative vaginal deliveries and the rate of cesarean deliveries for abnormal FHR patterns and/or acidosis.

INTRAPARTUM ASPHYXIA

Acute intrapartum hypoxia can lead to severe neonatal complications. In order to attribute an adverse neonatal outcome to intrapartum acidosis, four essential criteria must be met.

1. Evidence of metabolic acidosis in umbilical arterial cord blood sample (pH less than 7.00 and base deficit greater than or equal to 12 mEq /L)
2. Early onset of severe or moderate neonatal encephalopathy in infants born at 34 weeks' gestation or later
3. Cerebral palsy of the spastic quadriplegic or dyskinetic type
4. Exclusion of other etiologies such as trauma, coagulation disorders, infectious conditions, or genetic disorders

In addition, there needs to be an indication that the timing of the insult was intrapartum.

1. Sentinel hypoxic event occurring immediately before or during labor
2. Sudden and sustained fetal bradycardia or the absence of FHR variability in the presence of persistent late or variable decelerations, usually after a hypoxic sentinel event when the pattern previously was normal
3. Apgar scores of 0 to 3 beyond five minutes
4. Onset of multisystem involvement within 72 hours of birth
5. Early imaging study showing evidence of acute nonfocal cerebral abnormality

CATEGORIZATION OF FHR TRACINGS

The definition of a normal FHR tracing is a stable baseline rate within the normal range (110 to 160 bpm) with moderate variability. In 2008, the National Institute of Child Health and Human Development, the American College of Obstetricians and Gynecologists, and the Society for Maternal–Fetal Medicine sponsored a workshop on electronic FHR monitoring. This workshop established definitions for FHR interpretation and categorization as well as uterine activity, and categorized FHR patterns into three categories. The three-category system (Table 10.2—next page) provides a way to differentiate FHR tracings that require no specific intervention, those that require attention and possible resuscitative measures, and those that require immediate intervention and possible delivery.

Table 10.2: Classification of Categories of Fetal Heart Rate Tracings

Category I*	Category II†	Category III*

➢ Baseline rate between 110 to 160 beats per minutes (bpm)
➢ Moderate baseline variability
➢ Absent late or variable decelerations
➢ Presence or absence of early decelerations
➢ Presence or absence of accelerations
	➢ Bradycardia without absent baseline variability
	➢ Tachycardia
	➢ Minimal baseline variability
	➢ Absent baseline variability but without recurrent decelerations
	➢ Marked baseline variability
	➢ Absence of accelerations following fetal stimulation
	➢ Recurrent variable decelerations with minimal variability or moderate baseline variability
	➢ Prolonged deceleration lasting greater than or equal to two minutes but less than ten minutes
	➢ Recurrent late decelerations with moderate baseline variability
	➢ Variable decelerations associated with other characteristics such as slow return to baseline, "shoulders," or "overshoots"
		➢ Absent baseline variability associated with:
		  - Recurrent late decelerations
		  - Recurrent variable decelerations
		  - Bradycardia
		➢ Sinusoidal pattern

*These tracings include all of the following patterns.
†These tracings include but are not limited to the following patterns. Additionally, this category includes patterns not classified as Category I or III.
*These tracings include all of the following patterns.

Adapted from: Macones GA et al. (2008).

Figure 10.1: The FHR tracing can move between categories depending on the underlying fetal physiology and interventions of the care team

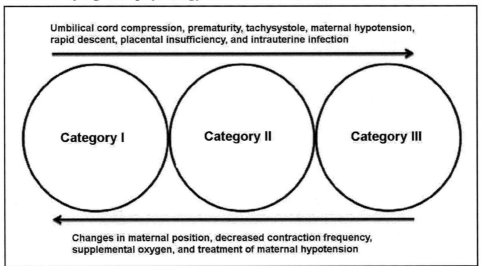

Umbilical cord compression, prematurity, tachysystole, maternal hypotension, rapid descent, placental insufficiency, and intrauterine infection

Category I   Category II   Category III

Changes in maternal position, decreased contraction frequency, supplemental oxygen, and treatment of maternal hypotension

INTERPRETATION OF FETAL HEART RATE TRACING CATEGORIES

Fetal heart rate tracing patterns provide information only on the current acid-base status of the fetus. As the physiology controlling FHR patterns is complex and fluid, an FHR tracing can change categories over time. In addition, the individual components of defined FHR patterns do not occur independently and generally evolve over time. Similarly, characteristics of FHR patterns are dependent upon fetal gestational age and physiologic status as well as maternal physiologic status. Thus, FHR tracings should be evaluated in the context of many clinical conditions including gestational age, prior results of fetal assessment, medications, maternal medical conditions, and fetal conditions (e.g., growth restriction, known congenital anomalies, fetal anemia, arrhythmia, etc.). The fetus can move between the different categories depending on the interventions performed by the care team to correct the fetal conditions and physiology underlying the tracing (Figure 10.1—previous page). Therefore, a Category III tracing secondary to maternal acidosis from diabetic ketoacidosis can resolve to a Category I after correction of maternal/fetal pathophysiology.

INTERVENTIONS

Based on the category of the FHR, certain interventions are recommended:

Category I FHR Tracings (Figure 10.2) are strongly predictive of normal fetal acid–base status at the time of observation. Category I FHR tracings may be monitored in a routine manner and no specific action is required.

Figure 10.2: Category I FHR Tracing

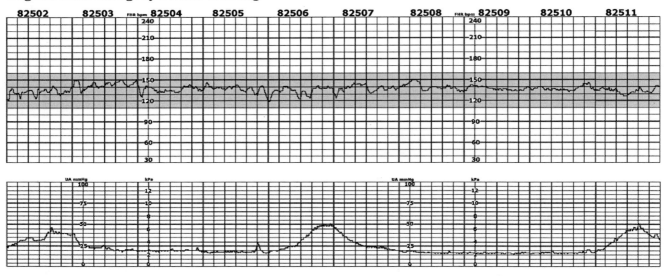

Category II FHR Tracings (Figure 10.3—next page) are indeterminate and are not predictive of abnormal fetal acid-base status but do require evaluation and continued surveillance. They are also the most common, occurring in the majority of fetuses in labor. The associated clinical circumstances, maternal conditions, medication exposures, fetal conditions, etc., should be taken into account. In some circumstances, either additional tests to ensure fetal well-being or intrauterine resuscitative measures may be used with Category II tracings. Recently, algorithms based on the presence of moderate variability and the presence of recurrent decelerations have

Figure 10.3: Category II FHR Tracing

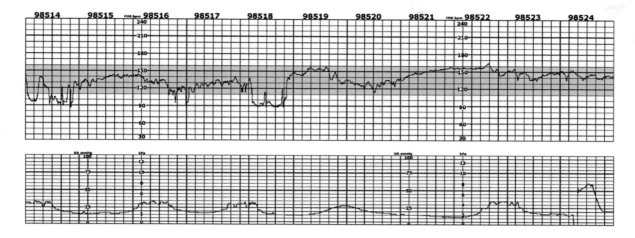

been proposed to assist in determining when delivery is indicated in the setting of a persistent Category II tracing. These algorithms have not yet been fully evaluated. Fetal pulse oximetry has not been shown to be clinically useful. Intrauterine resuscitation measures include discontinuation of any labor stimulating agent; cervical examination to rule out umbilical cord prolapse, rapid cervical dilation, or descent of the fetal head; changing maternal position to reduce compression of the vena cava and improve uteroplacental blood flow; monitoring maternal blood pressure and treatment with volume expansion or medications if warranted; and assessment and treatment of uterine **tachysystole.**

Category III FHR Tracings (Figure 10.4) are associated with abnormal fetal acid-base status at the time of observation. Category III FHR tracings require prompt evaluation. Depending on the clinical situation, efforts to expeditiously resolve the abnormal FHR pattern may include but are not limited to provision of maternal oxygen, change in maternal position, discontinuation of labor stimulation, treatment of maternal hypotension, and treatment of tachysystole. If a Category III tracing does not resolve with these measures, delivery should be undertaken.

Figure 10.4: Category III FHR Tracing

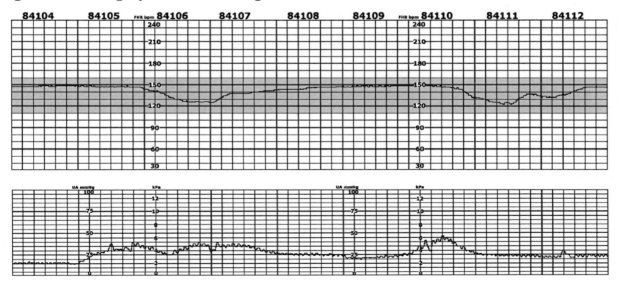

CONCLUSION

Fetal heart rate tracings during labor should be reviewed frequently by the healthcare team, approximately every 30 minutes in the active stage of labor and every 15 minutes during the second stage for uncomplicated patients. In patients with complications (e.g., fetal growth restriction, preeclampsia), review should be more frequent, every 15 minutes in the active stage of labor and every five minutes during the second stage. Healthcare providers periodically should document that they have reviewed the tracing. A full description of the EFM tracing requires a qualitative and quantitative description of uterine contractions, baseline FHR, baseline FHR variability, presence of accelerations, periodic or episodic decelerations, and changes or trends of FHR patterns over time. The FHR tracing should be maintained as part of the medical record and should be available for review in the future if needed.

RELATED READINGS

1. Association of Women's Health, Obstetric, and Neonatal Nurses (2015). Fetal Heart Rate Monitoring Principles and Practices (Ed. 5), Washington, D.C.: AWHONN.

2. American College of Obstetricians and Gynecologists (2010). Management of intrapartum fetal heart rate tracings. ACOG Practice Bulletin #116.

3. American College of Obstetricians and Gynecologists and American Academy of Pediatrics (2014). Neonatal encephalopathy and cerebral palsy: Defining the pathogenesis and pathophysiology (Ed 2).

4. American Academy of Pediatrics and American College of Obstetricians and Gynecologists (2017). Guidelines for Perinatal Care (Ed. 8).

5. Association of Women's Health, Obstetric, and Neonatal Nurses Practice Monograph (2013). Cervical Ripening and Induction and Augmentation of Labor (Ed. 4).

6. Clark SL, et al. (2013). Intrapartum management of category II fetal heart rate tracings: Towards standardization of care. American Journal of Obstetrics and Gynecology, 209(2):89-97.

7. Freeman RK, Garite TJ, and Nageotte MP (2003). Clinical management of nonreassuring fetal heart rate patterns (Chapter 9). Fetal Heart Rate Monitoring (Ed. 3). San Francisco, CA: Lippincott Williams and Wilkins, pp. 110-144 (see especially p. 129).

8. Garite TJ (2017). Intrapartum fetal evaluation (Chapter 15). IN: SG Gabbe, JR Niebyl, JL Simpson, et. al (Eds.) Obstetrics: Normal and Problem Pregnancies (Ed. 7), Philadelphia, PA: Churchill Livingston.

9. Macones GA, Hankins GDV, Spong CY, Hauth J, and Moore T (2008). The 2008 National Institute of Child Health and Human Development workshop report on electronic fetal monitoring: Update on definitions, interpretation, and research guidelines. American College of Obstetricians and Gynecologists, 112:661-666.

10. Thorp JM (2018). Clinical aspects of normal and abnormal labor (Chapter 36). In: R Resnik, CJ Lockwood, TR Moore, et. al (Eds.) Creasy and Resnik's Maternal-Fetal Medicine: Principles and Practice (Ed. 8), Philadelphia, PA: Saunders Elsevier.

Chapter 10 Review
Fetal Heart Rate Monitoring Interpretation

1. Your interpretation of an FHR tracing over a time span of 30 minutes is as follows:

    - Fetal heart rate baseline: 150 bpm
    - Fetal heart rate variability: Minimal (amplitude range greater than undetectable to less than or equal to 5 bpm)
    - Accelerations: Absent
    - Decelerations: Recurrent, late decelerations

    You would determine the FHR category of this tracing to be:

    A. Category I.
    B. Category II.
    C. Category III.

2. Maternal factors that can influence the fetus and cause changes in the FHR include:

    A. maternal respiratory status.
    B. placental condition.
    C. uteroplacental blood flow.
    D. cardiac output.
    E. all of the above.
    F. A, B, and D only.

3. Of the following FHR categories, the one(s) most reflective of an abnormal fetal acid-base status at the time of observation is:

    A. Category I.
    B. Category II.
    C. Category III.
    D. all of the above.
    E. B and C only.

4. When interpreting an FHR tracing, you note the presence of absent FHR baseline variability. You know the fetal acid-base balance at this time may be abnormal and the desired physiologic response(s) of your interventions is/are:

    A. an increase in available oxygen.
    B. an improvement in uteroplacental blood flow.
    C. an improvement in umbilical cord blood flow.
    D. an increase in maternal cardiac output.
    E. all of the above.
    F. A, B, and C only.

5. True or False. Accelerations must be present in a Category I tracing in order to indicate a normal fetal acid-base status.

    A. True
    B. False

Chapter 10 Review Answers
Fetal Heart Rate Monitoring Interpretation

1. **The correct answer is B.** The FHR variability is minimal (amplitude range greater than undetectable to less than or equal to 5 bpm), making this a Category II tracing. If it were absent it would be a Category III. However, this still is a very concerning tracing and warrants further assessment and interventions.

2. **The correct answer is E.** Any condition that causes an interruption in the availability of oxygen or perfusion of the uteroplacental unit will be reflected by changes in the fetal heart rate.

3. **The correct answer is C.** Category III tracings are more likely to be associated with abnormal fetal acid-base status; however, all the categories can be associated with both normal statuses depending on the clinical situation.

4. **The correct answer is E.**

5. **The correct answer is B.** Moderate FHR variability and normal FHR baseline rate indicate a normal fetal acid-base status.

Chapter 11

Fetal Assessment by Doppler Velocimetry

INTRODUCTION

The ability to assess fetal health from any single antenatal test is limited. Several antepartum fetal surveillance techniques/tests have been discussed previously in this text, including nonstress testing (NST), contraction stress testing (CST), and biophysical profile testing (BPP and modified BPP). Doppler assessment of vascular flow, especially umbilical artery Doppler velocimetry, has become an important part of full evaluation of the growth-restricted fetus and in making decisions regarding delivery.

The primary utility of Doppler is in the context of fetal growth restriction (FGR). The use of Doppler ultrasound in high-risk pregnancy has been shown in many trials to reduce the risk of perinatal deaths, and decrease the need for induction of labor and the risk of cesarean delivery. Thus, the available evidence suggests umbilical artery Doppler velocimetry can achieve better fetal and neonatal outcomes as primary antepartum surveillance based on results of the NST. If umbilical artery Doppler velocimetry is used, decisions regarding timing of delivery should be made using a combination of information from the Doppler ultrasonography, gestational age, and other tests of fetal status, such as amniotic fluid volume assessment, NST, CST, and BPP, along with careful monitoring of maternal condition.

Other fetal vessels with commonly used Doppler measurements include the middle cerebral artery, and fetal venous system with ductus venosus and umbilical vein. Doppler velocimetry of these fetal vessels can add to the management of fetal growth restriction, twin-to-twin transfusion syndrome, fetal anemia, and fetal cardiac function. For this chapter, however, we will concentrate primarily on the use of Doppler velocimetry in cases of FGR related to placental insufficiency, as well as Doppler testing relating to cases of suspected fetal anemia.

DOPPLER PRINCIPLE

Doppler ultrasonography provides information on vascular flow. The Doppler principle is based on the change in the frequency of reflected sound from a moving source. Whatever the initial frequency of the sound wave, motion of a reflecting object toward or away from a stationary object imparts a positive or negative component, adding or subtracting from the frequency, such that the pitch increases or decreases in accordance with the direction of movement. The most common example used to describe the Doppler shift is the change in the pitch of the sound of an approaching train to a stationary observer. The pitch increases as the train approaches and decreases as it travels away from the observer.

The same principle can be applied to a sound wave reflected from red blood cells flowing within a vessel. The faster the velocity of flow, the greater the Doppler shift. Accurate measurement of the peak velocity of flow is dependent on the angle of

Figure 11.1: Doppler Frequency Shift (DFS). Note that not only can the DFS be increased by increasing velocity, but it also can be increased by decreasing the angle (aligning the beam to the flow) or increasing the frequency of the sound waves.

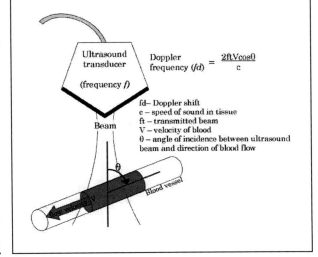

$$\text{Doppler frequency } (fd) = \frac{2ftV\cos\theta}{c}$$

fd – Doppler shift
c – speed of sound in tissue
ft – transmitted beam
V – velocity of blood
θ – angle of incidence between ultrasound beam and direction of blood flow

the transducer relative to the vessel, however. If the angle on insonation is 0° (i.e., if the transducer is exactly parallel to the vessel), the Doppler shift will correspond directly to velocity of flow. Any orientation other than *exactly parallel* to the vessel will underestimate flow; the extreme would be when the transducer is perpendicular to the vessel, in which case there will be no Doppler shift (and thus, no apparent flow), because the direction of flow is neither toward nor away from the transducer. When the angle is not 0°, there is a formula that allows those trigonometrically inclined to compensate based on the cosine of the angle (Figure 11.1—previous page).

The frequency shift of the ultrasound beam can be displayed in a time-frequency shift plot on the X and Y axis respectively. For arteries, the frequency shift will be highest at the peak speed, i.e., systole, and lowest at the nadir, i.e., at the end of diastole. For a given forward propulsive force, velocity of flow in the tissue is inversely proportional to impedance, and indirectly resistance to flow. Low resistance maximally facilitates forward flow during both systole and diastole, while higher resistance decreases both. By definition, systole reflects active forward propulsion, while diastole corresponds to passive flow. For this reason, a given increase in resistance will decrease diastolic flow more than systolic flow.

DOPPLER MEASUREMENT TECHNIQUES: DOPPLER RATIOS AND PEAK SYSTOLIC VELOCITY

All Doppler measurements should be performed in the absence of fetal breathing and body movements. Maternal movement and breathing movements also can affect the Doppler waveforms, and the mother should be asked to hold her breath during the recording. To obtain more accurate results, three to four measurements are done sequentially and then are averaged.

Doppler ultrasound enables us to measure volume flow and velocities. Actual volume of blood flow is difficult to measure and necessitates formulas

Table 11.1: Commonly Used Doppler Measurements

Peak Systolic Velocity (PSV): Maximum flow during systole

Systolic/Diastolic (S/D) Ratio: Ratio of peak systolic (S) to trough diastolic flow (D)

RI (resistance index) = $\dfrac{\text{S-D}}{\text{S}}$

PI (pulsatility index) = $\dfrac{\text{S-D}}{\text{Mean Velocity}}$

used in volume vessel diameters. Peak velocities should be assessed keeping the angle between the ultrasound beam and the flow as close to 0° as possible. Doppler ratios of different velocities of flow at various parts of an arterial or venous cycle give us an indirect estimation of resistance (impedance) to flow.

Doppler ratios are independent of the angle. For arteries, peak flow at systole (S) and peak flow at the end of diastole (D) or the mean flow throughout the cycle are used for calculating Doppler ratios. There are three such ratios, including:

- S/D (peak systolic flow/diastolic flow),
- RI (resistance index, $\dfrac{\text{S-D}}{\text{S}}$), and
- PI (pulsatility index, $\dfrac{\text{S-D}}{\text{Mean Velocity}}$).

The pulsatility index is a more reproducible index with the lowest margin of error and is recommended by many experts as the preferred ratio in clinical practice. It is also the only ratio that can be used in cases with no forward flow or reversed flow in diastole.

Figure 11.2: Umbilical Artery Doppler Waveform at 11, 25, and 34 Weeks.
Note the increase in diastolic flow (arrows) by gestational age.

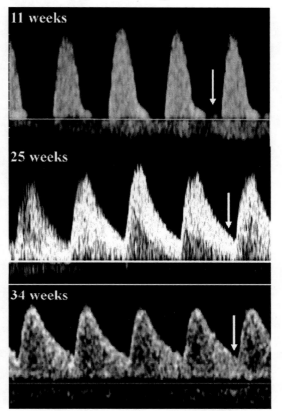

Many fetal blood vessels are accessible to Doppler velocimetry. In obstetrics, the umbilical artery (UA) is the most commonly assessed vessel. Routine measurement of UA Doppler in the low-risk population is not beneficial, but it is an important part of the evaluation and management of suspected FGR. Umbilical artery measurements should be performed at a free loop site. The ratios are reduced slightly at the placental insertion and the highest at the insertion to the fetal abdominal wall. The impact of the location of the measurement, however, clinically is not significant. The umbilical vein tracing may be helpful to rule out fetal breathing. Due to the gradual maturation of placental tertiary villi, there is an increase in diastolic flow with advancing gestation. Thus, in normal pregnancy, the Doppler ratios of the umbilical artery decrease as pregnancy progresses (Figure 11.2).

In pregnancies with placental insufficiency and related fetal growth restriction, the Doppler ratios of the umbilical artery remain elevated.

MIDDLE CEREBRAL ARTERY

The middle cerebral artery (MCA) is an easily visualized cerebral vessel with its straight course. It carries more than 80% of the cerebral blood flow. The vessel should be sampled soon after its origin from the internal carotid artery in the axial view of the circle of Willis. MCA Doppler waveform analysis can be used both for assessment of fetal anemia and to assess arterial redistribution in the growth-restricted fetus. In cases of fetal anemia, the peak systolic velocity (PSV) of MCA blood flow will be increased. PSV can be standardized as multiples of the median (MoM) for that gestational age. Moderate to severe anemia is much more likely when the MoM exceeds 1.5.

The growth-restricted fetus redistributes the blood flow to the vital organs including the brain, adrenals, and the coronary arteries. The increased supply of blood to the brain in hypoxemic fetuses is enabled by vasodilatation of intracerebral vessels. In Doppler velocimetry of human fetal MCA, this is reflected by the change in blood velocity waveforms with an increase in diastolic velocities and decreased Doppler ratios (increased flow). MCA can be visualized due to its straight course more easily then the adrenal and coronary arteries. Thus, decreased Doppler ratios of the MCA for FGR fetuses are consistent with so called "brain-sparing" effect in which blood preferentially is directed to the brain (see also Figure 11.6—page 143).

DOPPLER OF FETAL VEINS

Venous vessels in which Doppler studies often are performed include the umbilical vein (UV), ductus venosus (DV), and inferior vena cava (IVC). Umbilical vein flow typically is non-pulsatile, but the IVC and DV have undulating patterns due to atrial pressure-volume changes throughout the cardiac cycle. The IVC has notched forward flow except for brief backward flow during the atrial contraction.

Typically, IVC and most other veins have flow patterns with four phases: S is the systolic wave, which results from negative intraatrial pressure with movement of the atrioventricular septum toward the cardiac apex. The v wave is the result of positive intraatrial pressure created by overfilling of the right atrium. D is the diastolic wave, which results from negative intraatrial pressure caused by the opening of the tricuspid valve. The a wave reflects positive intraatrial pressure during atrial systole. F (Figure 11.3). The DV has a notched forward flow pattern, but normally, always should be forward unlike other veins that normally may have reversal of flow.

The DV is a slender trumpet-like shunt connecting the intra-abdominal umbilical vein to the inferior vena cava at its inlet to the heart and carries the most rapidly moving blood in the venous system. Under normal circumstances, the DV diverts 25% of umbilical venous flow toward the right atrium in this high-velocity stream, whereas 55% reach the left and 20% the right liver lobes. The DV flow is identifiable easily due to high velocity and resulting turbulent color flow on Doppler ultrasound. Oxygenated blood from the DV predominantly enters the left atrium via the foramen ovale, passes into the left ventricle and then out the aorta to supply the brain and the coronaries, i.e., so called "preferential streaming" (see Chapter 3 also). In normal fetuses, forward flow during atrial systole in DV increases with advancing gestational age (Figure 11.4).

Figure 11.3: Normal IVC Doppler Waveform.
Note the reversed flow during atrial systole (a). S, V, D, and a waves are noted.

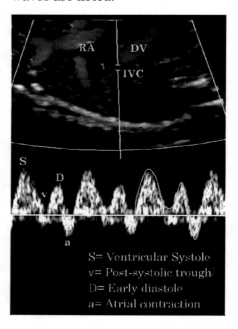

Figure 11.4: Normal DV Doppler Waveforms at 11, 24, and 33 Weeks.
Note, normally there is forward flow during atria systole (arrows) regardless of gestational age and it increases with gestational age. The S, v, D, and a waves are noted in the final tracing.

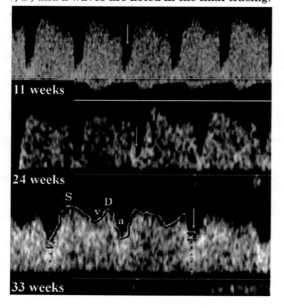

SUSPECTED FETAL ANEMIA AND MIDDLE CEREBRAL ARTERY DOPPLER

Fetal anemia can have many causes (e.g., Rh or other alloimmunizations, parvovirus infection, hemoglobin-opathies, fetomaternal hemorrhage, or twin-to-twin transfusion syndrome). In severe cases, fetal anemia can lead to cardiac failure and hydrops. Fortunately, Doppler ultrasound can help avoid delaying diagnosis until this point by providing a noninvasive method to assess for fetal anemia.

The peak systolic MCA peak systolic Doppler velocity (MCA PSV) is a reliable noninvasive screening tool to detect fetal anemia. Fetal anemia results in "thin" blood with less oxygen-carrying capacity than normal. The fetus attempts to compensate for this by increasing cardiac output to maintain oxygen delivery, thereby increasing the velocity of blood flow to the brain. Middle cerebral artery PSV is increased in fetal anemia due to enhanced fetal cardiac output and a decrease in blood viscosity. Since MCA velocity

140

increases with advancing gestational age, results are reported in multiples of the median (MoM) for that particular gestational age much like maternal serum alpha fetoprotein (MSAFP).

In the follow up of Rh or other alloimmunizations, MCA PSV has the advantage of being a noninvasive test. In the not-so-distant past, identification of the alloimmunized anemic fetus has involved invasive methods such as serial amniocentesis that measured the bilirubin levels. In most alloimmunized fetuses, fetal red blood cells are destroyed by the fetal spleen once maternal antibodies are bound to the cell causing fetal anemia and hemolysis. Bilirubin is the product of hemolysis and levels can be measured in the amniotic fluid by a spectrophometric test that is called delta PD450, to indirectly indicate the severity of anemia. Now, Doppler for MCA PSV provides a noninvasive alternative. It also has been shown that MCA PSV is more sensitive and accurate than the conventional and invasive testing of delta OD_{450} levels without the necessity of amniocentesis. Patients above the critical titers or with history of previously affected fetuses can have serial MCA PSV testing starting as early as 16 weeks' gestation instead of amniocentesis. Initial follow up should be by weekly assessments. Depending on the slope of increase and the initial titer level, measurements can be performed every one to two weeks. A value of greater than 1.5 MoM is used as a cutoff to diagnose moderate to severe anemia and is an indication for percutaneous blood sampling to investigate for fetal anemia and intrauterine blood transfusion as needed. MCA PSV can be falsely positive after 35 weeks' gestation, however, and positive results should be interpreted with caution. In these cases, delivery may be considered after a course of steroids.

FETAL GROWTH RESTRICTION

Fetal growth restriction occurs when some pathologic process interferes with a fetus fulfilling its growth potential. Fetal weight can be estimated by ultrasound by using various measurements such as head circumference, biparietal diameter, abdominal circumference, and femur length into a formula. Estimated fetal weight (EFW) then can be compared to others at that gestational age, typically using percentiles. Fetal growth restriction is suspected when an EFW is below the 10th percentile for gestational age or an abdominal circumference is less than the 5th percentile. Placental insufficiency (intrinsic or due to maternal vascular disease), genetic abnormalities, infection, structural anomalies, and various syndromes all are associated with FGR. It can be difficult to distinguish the constitutionally small fetus (smaller than usual but otherwise normal) from the growth-restricted fetus, however, and timing and onset of the growth delay, maternal history, and associated ultrasound findings can be helpful in establishing an etiology. Because the most common reason for FGR is placental insufficiency, umbilical artery Doppler velocimetry can be valuable in making this determination.

The terminology surrounding FGR can be confusing. Textbooks often define FGR as an EFW less than the 10th percentile for gestational age, analogous to calling any birthweight less than the 10th percentile "small for gestational age" (SGA). In fact, most fetuses with EFW less than the 10th percentile are not growth-restricted; they are normal, constitutionally small fetuses that just happen to fall below an arbitrary threshold. It would be clearer if an EFW less than the 10th percentile was called SGA, with subsequent investigation and monitoring to determine whether such a fetus actually is growth restricted. This is where umbilical artery Doppler comes in handy. Abnormalities in diastolic blood flow through the umbilical artery often constitute the first sign of FGR after diagnosis of an SGA fetus. Other vascular manifestations of placental dysfunction that aid in the diagnosis include:

1.   Increased uterine artery Doppler index and/or notching.
2.   Decreased middle cerebral artery Doppler ratios.

3. Decreased cerebroplacental Doppler index ratios, for example decreased MCA-PI:UA-PI.
4. Amniotic fluid index less than 5 cm.

PRECLINICAL SIGNS OF PLACENTAL DYSFUNCTION: VENOUS REDISTRIBUTION

One of the earliest signs of placental dysfunction is decreased umbilical venous volume flow. Before umbilical artery Doppler becomes abnormal, reduced umbilical venous volume flow leads to the reduction of the proportion of fetal cardiac output distributed to the placenta and to increased DV shunting blood away from the liver and towards the heart. This venous redistribution is associated with down regulation of the glucose-insulin-IgF growth axis and decreased glycogen store in the liver. Therefore, decreased abdominal circumference due to decreased liver size is the first clinical sign of lagging fetal growth before the composite estimated fetal weight falls below the 10th percentile.

EARLY SIGNS OF FGR: ARTERIAL REDISTRIBUTION

The placental circulation normally is very low resistance, because there is no reason why fetal blood should have difficulty traversing the villi to gain oxygen and nutrients while eliminating waste. When the placental function is abnormal, from the shallow/incomplete invasion and/or incomplete formation of the low-resistance tertiary villi, however, the total cross-sectional area of available villous capillaries is decreased. This leads to increased vascular resistance, and changes in the arterial Doppler waveforms.

UMBILICAL ARTERY DOPPLER

Umbilical artery Doppler ratio measurements help differentiate constitutionally small fetuses from FGR due to placental insufficiency and aid in monitoring FGR. As mentioned earlier, increased downstream resistance in a poorly functioning placenta preferentially affects passive diastolic flow more than it does active systolic flow. Diastolic blood flow continues to decrease, and may eventually stop with increased placental compromise, and in cases of extremely high resistance, may even be reflected backwards in what is called reversed end-diastolic flow (Figure 11.5). A decrease in umbilical artery end-diastolic velocity and an increase in Doppler ratios develop once 30% or more of the placental villous vasculature is abnormal. Once 60% to 70% of the villous tree is damaged, absent or reversed end-diastolic flow (AEDF/REDF) occurs. Serial measurements of Doppler indices of the umbilical artery help us understand the nature and severity of FGR and enable us to better manage it, especially when preterm.

Figure 11.5: Absent and Reversed End Diastolic Flow (arrows) in the Umbilical Artery

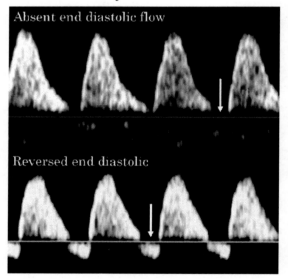

Absent end diastolic flow

Reversed end diastolic

MIDDLE CEREBRAL ARTERY DOPPLER

The growth-restricted fetus redistributes the blood flow to the vital organs including the brain, adrenals, and coronary arteries. For the brain, this involves lowering resistance by vasodilation in the cerebral arteries to improve blood flow and oxygen delivery, leading to decreased MCA Doppler ratios, i.e., the "brain-sparing" effect (Figure 11.6). Decreases in MCA Doppler ratios suggest preferential perfusion of the brain by autoregulation. Early subclinical elevation of placental vascular resistance, along with decreasing resistance in the cerebral circulation, produce an increase in umbilical artery and a decrease in the middle cerebral artery Doppler ratios. The so-called cerebroplacental ratio, or MCA RI/UA PI becomes abnormal, measuring above 1.1.

As the placental function continues to decline, the Doppler ratios will continue to change to reflect this redistribution.

Figure 11.6: Middle Cerebral Artery Doppler Waveforms Showing Both Normal and Brain Sparing Physiology.
Note the relative increased flow during diastole (arrows) resulting in a lower MCA PI.

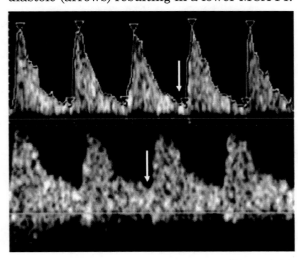

DUCTUS VENOSUS DOPPLER

Figure 11.7: Abnormal DV Dopplers.
Note: Absent flow velocity (arrow) during atrial systole in ductus venosus Doppler

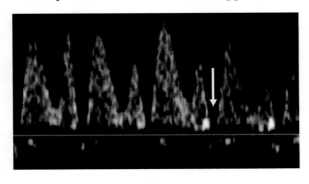

The DV is responsible for shunting oxygen-rich blood from the umbilical vein to the right heart. As the fetus grows, demand increases, with increasing forward DV flow during atrial systole with advancing gestational age (Figure 11.4—page 140). In cases with FGR due to abnormal placentation, fetuses develop a higher degree of DV shunting of umbilical venous flow, probably as a redistributional adaptation to hypoxemia, ensuring oxygenation of the heart and brain. Therefore, an absence or reversal of DV flow during atrial systole is highly concerning and currently is thought of as the last stage of fetal cardiovascular deterioration and, therefore, a high risk of fetal death (Figure 11.7).

LATE SIGNS OF FGR: CRITICAL DOPPLERS AND BIOPHYSICAL PROFILE SCORE ABNORMALITIES

Signs of accelerating placental dysfunction and worsening fetal status include:

1. Umbilical artery absent or reversed end-diastolic velocity (AEDF/REDF)
2. MCA Doppler evidence of brain sparing
3. Elevated venous Doppler ratios
4. Reversal of ductus venosus atrial wave
5. Umbilical vein pulsations

6. Oligohydramnios
7. Abnormal biophysical profile score

When villous obliteration affects 50% to 70% of the placenta, umbilical artery end diastolic flow velocity may be absent or reversed with a proportionally increased risk for fetal hypoxemia and/or acidemia (Figure 11.8). This marked increase of placental blood flow resistance translates into higher aortic blood pressures, making it more difficult for blood to flow through the ductus arteriosus. Secondary right ventricular afterload results in shunting towards the left ventricle and increased left ventricular output.

Simultaneously, the increase in placental vascular resistance causes a decrease in the forward diastolic blood flow through the aortic isthmus. With further deterioration, reverse blood flow occurs, in which blood coming from the pulmonary artery and descending aorta is diverted from the placenta to the brain. Although cerebral blood flow is increased, the brain is perfused partly by blood that is deprived of substrates essential for fetal development and, at the same time, by red blood cells poorly saturated with oxygen.

Figure 11.8: Sequence of Doppler Abnormalities in Early-Onset FGR

Placental Dysfunction
⇩
Venous Redistribution
(Decreased UV flow)
⇩
Arterial Redistribution
(MCA RI/UA RI >1.1)
⇩
Placental Resistance Increases
⇩
Umbilical Arterial Flow Abnormal
(Elevation UA ratio, AEDF/REDF)
⇩
Further Arterial Redistribution
(MCA PI low)
⇩
Venous Flow Abnormal
(DV notching, UV pulsations)
⇩
Fetal Demise

Abnormalities in the fetal venous system occur late in the process (Figure 11.8). Marked DV dilation to increase cardiac diversion of umbilical venous blood leads to increased retrograde transmission of the atrial pressure and volume changes. A decline in cardiac performance contributes to an elevation of central venous pressure and decreasing forward cardiac function. Under these circumstances, a-wave reversal in the DV and progressive pulsatility in the umbilical vein is observed. Hepatic artery dilation provides evidence for an attempt to counteract the hepatic seal from excessive venous shunting by increasing the arterial contribution to liver blood supply.

As progressive arterial and venous Doppler abnormalities accelerate, fetal biophysical parameters are lost in a sequential manner determined by the relative sensitivity of the central regulatory centers to hypoxemia. Loss of fetal heart rate reactivity precedes loss of breathing, gross body movements, and tone. Decreasing amniotic fluid volume is independent of biophysical progression, a later sign of chronic hypoxemia more closely related to cardiovascular deterioration (Figure 11.9).

Figure 11.9: Sequence of Loss of Fetal Biophysical Profile Parameters in FGR as pH Declines

Reactive NST
⇩
Loss of Fetal Heart Rate Reactivity
⇩
Loss of Breathing
⇩
Loss of Gross Body Movements
⇩
Loss of Fetal Tone
⇩
Death

Note: Decreasing amniotic fluid volume is independent of BPP progression; it is more closely related to cardiovascular deterioration than to pH status

144

The above sequence of cardiovascular events and reflective Doppler changes apply to the early-onset FGR prior to 34 weeks. In early-onset FGR with elevated umbilical artery Doppler ratios but positive end-diastolic velocity, the overall perinatal mortality is 5.6%. This percentage increases to 11.5% when end-diastolic velocity is absent or reversed but venous Doppler indices still are normal. Perinatal mortality increases almost four-fold to 38.8% when venous Doppler indices (DV, UV) become abnormal, predominantly because of an increase in the rate of stillbirths.

Fetal surveillance frequency can be adjusted taking into account the fetal interval growth, cardiac parameters, Doppler changes, and amniotic fluid volume. In early-onset FGR, safe prolongation of pregnancy is a primary goal, whereas recognizing the subtle features of progressive compromise appears to be the major challenge of term FGR. In the presence of positive umbilical artery end diastolic velocity, clinical deterioration is unlikely to occur within one week. Absent or reversed end-diastolic flow (AEDF/REDF) in the umbilical artery and increasing DV Doppler ratios should lead to frequent monitoring (more than once weekly) or hospital admission with daily monitoring. Reversal of the DV a-wave increases the risk for an abnormal biophysical profile score within one to eight days, and at least daily testing is recommended.

USE OF DOPPLER VELOCIMETRY FOR TIMING OF DELIVERY IN EARLY-ONSET FGR

In early-onset FGR, gestational age and birth weight are the primary determinants of outcome, especially before 28 weeks. While early intervention carries a high risk of neonatal prematurity-related complications and increased neonatal mortality, delayed delivery is associated with an increased risk of stillbirth. However, each day gained *in utero* increases survival and intact survival by 1% to 2% with the highest gain between 24 to 28 weeks' gestation. Thereafter, survival benefits per day decline and thresholds for delivery may be lower.

At present, there is no randomized treatment trial on the performance of specific monitoring regimens and delivery triggers in improving outcomes in FGR. The traditional assumption about long-term fetal impact of placental disease was that fetal metabolic deterioration precedes abnormal neurodevelopment and that early intervention could modify this cascade. However, recent data suggests that by the time FGR clinically is apparent, many fetal organs (including the brain) already have been subjected to abnormal blood flow and nutrient supply. Thus, fetal neurodevelopment is affected already before the cascade of fetal deterioration is evident, and changing delivery timing is unlikely to change many aspects of long-term neurodevelopmental outcome. Therefore, the goals of care are prevention of stillbirth and maximization of gestational age.

Available studies suggest that lagging head circumference, overall degree of FGR, gestational age, and umbilical artery, aortic, and cerebral Doppler parameters are independent prenatal determinants of infant and childhood neurodevelopment. Head circumference as well is an important metric and is independent of gestational age; the degree of FGR has the greatest impact on this metric when there is early-onset FGR. Gestational age has an overriding negative effect on neurodevelopment until 32 to 34 weeks' gestation. For the umbilical artery and aorta, the developmental impact is proportional to the degree of decrease in end-diastolic velocity, with the worst outcomes if REDF develops by 27 weeks' gestation.

Observational and management studies do not suggest that further fetal deterioration (e.g., abnormal venous Doppler indices or worsening BPP) has an independent impact on neurodevelopment in early-onset FGR. In clinical practice, immediate delivery greater than or equal to 32 weeks with REDF in the umbilical artery and greater than or equal to 34 weeks with AEDF in the umbilical artery is suggested. DV Doppler indices can be used after 27 to 28 weeks to support expectant management if normal and can guide the need for closer monitoring due to a higher risk of perinatal death if severely abnormal.

In an effort to clarify the optimum timing by prenatal testing, the TRUFFLE study in Europe randomized women with singleton fetuses at 26 to 32 weeks' gestation with FGR and a high umbilical artery Doppler index (greater than the 95th percentile) to three timing of delivery plans, which differed according to antenatal monitoring strategies: reduced short-term variability by cardiotocography (CTG STV), elevated ductus venosus (DV) Doppler ratios greater than the 95th percentile and reversed a wave in the DV. The proportion of infants surviving without neuroimpairment was similar among the three groups. Of survivors, more infants in the reversed a wave DV changes group were free of neuroimpairment; however, this was accompanied by a non-significant increase in perinatal and infant mortality. The authors concluded between 26 to 32 weeks' gestation, a conservative approach to timing delivery in waiting for late ductus venosus changes is associated with a more favorable two-year outcome. However, the authors used a strategy of safety net CTG changes that overrode randomization and led to delivery. Given this "safety CTG net approach" and the use of computer-based CTG that is not widely available, the reproducibility and generalization to other populations remain unclear.

In summary, the optimal timing of delivery in early-onset FGR is unknown and, as mentioned above, much of the neurodevelopmental impact on the fetus likely occurs before clinical presentation is apparent. A conservative approach may be considered prior to 32 weeks' gestation in order to reduce neuroimpairment with the caveat that fetal death rate may be increased.

Most importantly, prevention of FGR, when possible, by optimization of maternal medical status, smoking cessation, and maximization of nutrition is the ideal strategy.

USE OF DOPPLER VELOCIMETRY FOR TIMING OF DELIVERY IN LATE-ONSET FGR

Late-onset FGR after 34 weeks is a significant clinical problem that contributes to over 50% of unanticipated stillbirths at term. Late FGR is characterized by few Doppler abnormalities and subtle biophysical findings suggesting fetal jeopardy. Elevated umbilical artery Doppler ratios are not common because the tertiary villi of the placenta already have developed before this late onset process starts. Isolated brain sparing, decreased cerebroplacental ratio (MCA RI/ UA RI less than 1.1), and loss of fetal heart rate reactivity are characteristic abnormalities in these patients. In this group of FGR fetuses, changes in cerebral artery resistance are associated with behavioral, psychologic, and cognitive abnormalities.

In the late-onset FGR fetus, prematurity risks are decreased, and the risk of fetal demise becomes the primary concern. There are no randomized trials addressing the timing of delivery of the late-onset FGR fetus. Timing the delivery of the late preterm/early-term FGR fetus requires consideration of multiple factors including degree of growth restriction, etiology, amniotic fluid volume, and BPP and Doppler testing. Available data suggests that delivery should occur by 37 to 38 weeks for singleton FGR fetuses with normal testing and earlier with significant FGR and associated oligohydramnios or well-being testing abnormalities.

RELATED READINGS

1. American College of Obstetricians and Gynecologists (1999). Antepartum fetal surveillance. <u>ACOG Practice Bulletin #9</u>.

2. Baschat AA (2010). Fetal growth restriction: From observation to intervention. <u>Journal of Perinatal Medicine</u>, 38:239–246.

3. Baschat A (2011). Neurodevelopment following fetal growth restriction and its relationship with antepartum parameters of placental dysfunction. <u>Ultrasound in Obstetrics and Gynecology</u>, 37: 501–514.

4. Baschat AA (2011). Venous Doppler evaluation of the growth-restricted fetus. <u>Clinics in Perinatology</u>, 38:103–112.

5. Baschat AA, Cosmi E, Bilardo CM, Wolf H, Berg C, Rigano S, Germer U, Moyano D, Turan S, Hartung J, Bhide A, Müller T, Bower S, Nicolaides KM, Thilaganathan B, Gembruch U, Ferrazzi E, Hecher K, Galan HL, and Harman CR (2007). Predictors of neonatal outcome in early-onset placental dysfunction. <u>Obstetrics and Gynecology</u>, 109:253–261.

6. Baschat AA and Odibo AO (2011). Timing of delivery in fetal growth restriction and childhood development: Some uncertainties remain. <u>American Journal of Obstetrics and Gynecology</u>, 204(1):2-3.

7. Bilardo CM, Wolf H, Stigter RH, Ville Y, Baez E, Visser GH, and Hecher K (2004). Relationship between monitoring parameters and perinatal outcome in severe, early intrauterine growth restriction. <u>Ultrasound in Obstetrics and Gynecology</u>, 23:119–125.

8. Camille Hoffman and Henry L. Galan (2009). Assessing the 'at-risk' fetus: Doppler ultrasound. <u>Current Opinion in Obstetrics and Gynecology</u>, 21:161–166.

9. Eixarch E, Meler E, Iraola A, Illa M, Crispi F, Hernandez- Andrade E, Gratacos E, and Figueras F (2008). Neurodevelopmental outcome in 2-year-old infants who were small-for-gestational age term fetuses with cerebral blood flow redistribution. <u>Ultrasound in Obstetrics and Gynecology</u>, 32:894–899.

10. Galan HL (2011). Timing delivery of the growth-restricted fetus. <u>Seminars in Perinatology</u>, 35:262-269.

11. Giles WB, Trudinger BJ, and Baird PJ (1985). Fetal umbilical artery flow velocity waveforms and placental resistance: Pathological correlation. <u>British Journal of Obstetrics and Gynaecology</u>, 92:31–38.

12. GRIT Study Group (2003). A randomized trial of timed delivery for the compromised preterm fetus: Short term outcomes and Bayesian interpretation. <u>British Journal of Obstetrics and Gynaecology</u>, 110:27-32.

13. Kiserud T (2005). Physiology of the fetal circulation. <u>Seminars in Fetal & Neonatal Medicine</u>, 10(6):493-503.

14. Lees C and Baumgartner H (2005). The TRUFFLE study: A collaborative publicly funded project from concept to reality: How to negotiate an ethical, administrative and funding obstacle course in the European Union. Ultrasound in Obstetrics and Gynecology, 25:105–107.

15. Lees CC, Marlow N, van Wassenaer-Leemhuis A, Arabin B, Bilardo CM, Brezinka C (2015). Two-year neurodevelopmental and intermediate perinatal outcomes in infants with very preterm fetal growth restriction (TRUFFLE): A randomized trial. Lancet, 30, 385(9983):2162-72.

16. Mari G, Deter RL, Carpenter RL, Rahman F, Zimmerman R, Moise Jr KJ, Dorman KF, Ludomirsky A, Gonzalez R, Oz U, Detti L, Copel JA, Bahado-Singh R, Berry S, Martinez-Poyer J, and Blackwell SC (2000). Noninvasive diagnosis by Doppler ultrasonography of fetal anemia due to maternal red-cell alloimmunization: Collaborative group for Doppler assessment of the blood velocity in anemic fetuses. New England Journal of Medicine, 342:9-14.

17. Miller J, Turan S, and Baschat AA (2008). Fetal growth restriction. Seminars in Perinatology, 32:274-280.

18. Morrow RJ, Adamson SL, Bull SB, and Ritchie AW (1989). Effect of placental embolization on the umbilical arterial velocity waveform in fetal sheep. American Journal of Obstetrics and Gynecology, 161:1055–1060.

19. Oepkes D, Seaward PG, Vandenbussche FP, Windrim R, Kingdom J, Beyene J, Kanhai HH, Ohlsson A, Ryan G, and DIAMOND Study Group (2006). Doppler ultrasonography versus amniocentesis to predict fetal anemia. New England Journal of Medicine, 355(2):156-164.

20. Roza SJ, Steegers EA, Verburg BO, Jaddoe VW, Moll HA, Hofman A, Verhulst FC, and Tiemeier H (2008). What is spared by fetal brain-sparing? Fetal circulatory redistribution and behavioral problems in the general population. American Journal of Epidemiology, 168:1145–1152.

21. Vossbeck S, de Camargo OK, Grab D, Bode H, and Pohlandt F (2001). Neonatal and neurodevelopmental outcome in infants born before 30 weeks of gestation with absent or reversed end diastolic flow velocities in the umbilical artery. European Journal of Pediatrics, 160:128–134.

22. Walker DM, Marlow N, Upstone L, Gross H, Hornbuckle J, Vail A, Wolke D, and Thornton JG (2011). The growth restriction intervention trial: Long-term outcomes in a randomized trial of timing of delivery in fetal growth restriction. American Journal of Obstetrics and Gynecology, 204(1):34.e1-9. Epub 2010 Nov 5.

Chapter 11 Review

Fetal Assessment by Doppler Velocimetry

1. Fetal growth restriction (FGR) is a term applied to a fetus with an abdominal circumference less than ____ or an estimated fetal weight below the ____ for its gestational age.

    A. 5th percentile; 1st percentile
    B. 5th percentile; 10th percentile
    C. 5th percentile; 5th percentile
    D. 10th percentile; 10th percentile

2. The etiology of FGR fetuses may be attributed to:

    A. chronic hypertension.
    B. maternal renal disease.
    C. aneuploidies.
    D. all of the above.
    E. A and C only.

3. True or False. Doppler velocimetry has been shown to have predictive value for fetal outcome in FGR fetuses.

    A. True
    B. False

4. Middle cerebral artery Dopplers can be used to assess for fetal anemia, as well as to check for:

    A. venous return to the heart from the brain.
    B. reduced perfusion of the fetal brain.
    C. increased perfusion to the fetal brain.
    D. evidence of brain damage in the fetus.

5. The correct sequence of loss of fetal biophysical profile parameters in FGR as pH declines is:

    A. reactive nonstress test → loss of gross body movements → loss of breathing.
    B. loss of gross body movements → loss of fetal tone → reactive nonstress test.
    C. decreased amniotic fluid → loss of gross body movements → loss of fetal tone.
    D. reactive nonstress test → loss of breathing → loss of gross body movements.

Chapter 11 Review Answers
Fetal Assessment by Doppler Velocimetry

1.   The correct answer is B.

2.   The correct answer is D.

3.   The correct answer is A.

4.   The correct answer is C.

5.   The correct answer is D.

Chapter 12

Fetal Monitoring in the Complex Patient

INTRODUCTION

Although fetal heart rate (FHR) monitoring is important in assessing fetal oxygenation status during pregnancy and labor, it is not always possible to obtain continuous, reliable FHR tracings. There are a number of maternal and fetal conditions that make FHR monitoring difficult, and sometimes multiple maternal and fetal conditions co-exist, challenging one's ability to effectively monitor at all. This chapter discusses these challenges and how to manage them.

INFECTION AND INTRAPARTUM FETAL HEART RATE MONITORING

In general, fetal monitoring should be done externally unless an adequate FHR tracing cannot be obtained. Internal monitoring may be very helpful in assessing the fetus when the external tracing is technically difficult to obtain or the variability of the baseline is decreased. However, there are some patients in whom internal FHR monitoring should be avoided.

For patients with hepatitis C and/or human immunodeficiency virus (HIV), internal FHR monitoring may increase the chance of transmission to the fetus and should be avoided when possible. The transmission rate of hepatitis C virus (HCV) from mother to fetus is negligible when the mother has HCV antibodies but is RNA-negative. When HCV antibodies are present with HCV RNA, the rate of vertical transmission is 4.2 to 7.8%. The rate rises to 7.6 to 15.2% with concurrent HIV infection (Benova, 2014). It is plausible that a break in fetal skin from a fetal scalp electrode could provide access for the virus. Although the evidence is conflicting, some studies have reported an increased risk of transmission with FHR internal monitoring. The general recommendation, therefore, is that providers avoid internal monitoring in these patients if at all possible. Similarly, for those mothers with HIV that are planning vaginal delivery (viral loads less than 1,000 copies/mL), internal monitoring should also be avoided. Although the risk of transmission of HIV is small when viral loads are low (approximately 2%) and is likely due to transplacental infection preceding labor, it is possible that placement of a fetal scalp electrode might increase this risk. The available data are limited, but the benefits of internal FHR monitoring in the setting of HCV and/or HIV infection may not be worth the possibly increased risk of vertical transmission.

MATERNAL OBESITY

With more than 1.6 billion overweight adults worldwide, obesity is a major contributor to the global burden of chronic disease and disability. Obese women are at higher risk for poor perinatal outcomes, which can range from shoulder dystocia to fetal death; thus, fetal monitoring is of great importance in these patients. However, fetal monitoring in severely obese patients often presents a technical challenge.

When positioning a severely obese patient, pillows, rolled blankets, and wedges may help improve patient comfort and maximize the success of fetal monitoring. Bariatric beds can make patient positioning easier, as can the use of Hoyer lifts and hover mats. Care should be taken to ensure that equipment has been assessed for weight limits (including operative tables) and that door widths will accommodate bariatric beds in the event of an emergency requiring swift transport. Toilets and commodes should be reinforced as needed. Staff should work collaboratively to create a care plan that identifies potential challenges for severely obese patients and all care providers should be made situationally aware.

If difficulty due to maternal habitus is encountered when attempting to continuously monitor FHR, ultrasound can be used to determine the optimal location for transducer placement. Rolled washcloths can be used to obtain optimal transducer angles. Particularly challenging cases may require handholding the transducer until a complete tracing can be obtained. If fetal monitoring straps are not long enough to secure transducers comfortably, longer straps should be used. Tying straps together should be avoided, because knots may shift, causing patient discomfort, pressure, bruising, and skin breakdown. If continuous monitoring is unsuccessful, FHR assessment can be attempted with intermittent auscultation. If the amniotic membranes are ruptured (or can be ruptured) during labor, there should be a low threshold for applying a fetal scalp electrode if the external monitor is not tracing well.

For uterine contraction assessment, the tocodynamometer should be placed on the thinnest portion of the abdomen so that uterine contractions are transmitted well. The tocodynamometer should be secured such that it lays flat on the abdomen, avoiding skin folds where it will be prone to tipping and/or flipping. If a pannus is present, the abdominal contours may be such that the uterus is actually quite high relative to the umbilicus. Palpation or ultrasound marking of the fundus may be helpful. Assessing uterine contractions can be especially difficult in the obese preterm patient, and certainly, these are the patients for whom accurate assessment is most crucial. If difficulty is encountered, it may be necessary to assess the frequency and duration of uterine contractions by palpation alone. Again, during the intrapartum period there should be a low threshold for using an intrauterine pressure catheter (IUPC) after rupture of membranes to assess timing or strength of contractions in relation to FHR patterns.

MULTIPLE GESTATION

Multiple gestation—particularly higher-order multiples—present a special challenge when it comes to fetal monitoring. Not only are there more fetuses to contend with, but maternal habitus is significantly altered. Additionally, patients carrying more than one fetus often experience more frequent discomfort, limiting their ability to sit or lie in fixed positions for extended periods of time. For this reason, adequate monitoring in these patients may prove difficult. To accommodate maternal movement, holding one or more of the monitors by hand may be required.

It is important that women with multiple gestations are positioned optimally before starting FHR monitoring. Vena caval compression and supine hypotension are more likely in multiple gestations and, therefore, maternal lateral tilt is essential. Ultrasound marking of fetal heart positions can be helpful and, in some situations, simultaneous recording of the maternal heart rate can help distinguish it from the FHRs. Baseline FHRs are often very similar and, as movement of one fetus often stimulates the others, tend to accelerate in concert. This can make it difficult to discern the FHR of baby A from that of baby B, and so on. It, therefore, is essential that all fetuses be monitored simultaneously to ensure that each is being monitored independently.

PREMATURITY

In general, a preterm fetus is monitored in the same way as a term fetus. It is the interpretation of the FHR tracing that differs based on gestational age. A neurologically immature preterm fetus may exhibit a higher baseline heart rate, particularly in the periviable and early preterm period. Small variable decelerations are common and rarely consequential. Although a preterm fetus may manifest accelerations that rise to 15 beats above baseline, these occur less frequently than at term. For nonstress testing (NST) in the fetus before 32 weeks, accelerations only need be ten beats above baseline for ten seconds ("10-by-10") to meet criteria for reactivity (Figure 12.1—next page). It also is important to understand that the premature fetus may exhibit 15-by-15 accelerations on one occasion and 10-by-10 accelerations on the next occasion, and that the

Figure 12.1: A Fetus 26 Weeks' Gestation Undergoing Nonstress Testing with Ten-Beat Criteria Accelerations, which is Normal for this Gestational Age

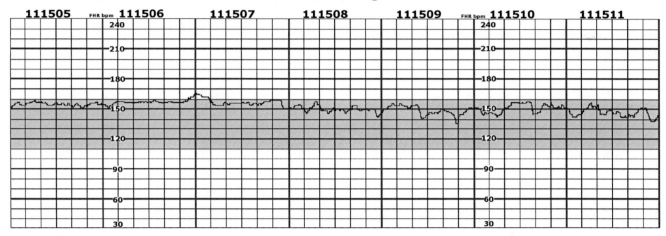

Figure 12.2: Preterm Infant at 27 Weeks Before and After Magnesium Sulfate Administration. Note the profound effects from magnesium sulfate on baseline FHR variability.

Before magnesium sulfate

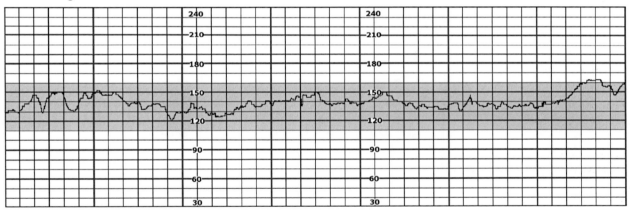

After magnesium sulfate

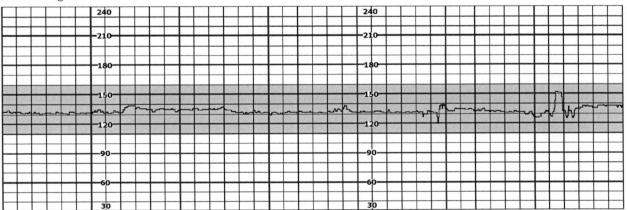

varying degree of reactivity does not change the outcome or interpretation of the test. Just because a preterm fetus was reactive with accelerations meeting 15-by-15 criteria on one occasion does not mean that it has to meet this criterion on all future nonstress tests before 32 weeks. Regardless, a reactive NST has similar predictive values in preterm and term pregnancies, correlating with a non-hypoxemic fetus. In preterm pregnancies, the criterion used for NST interpretation is much less important to outcomes than the gestational age at delivery. There are no appreciable differences between the ten-beat criteria and 15-beat criteria in predicting outcome, and therefore, for fetuses less than 32 weeks, the ten-beat criteria are sufficient (Glantz, 2011).

During intrapartum monitoring of the preterm fetus, it is important to anticipate the reduced variability at baseline and more pronounced reductions in variability in response to sleep states, stress, and medications, especially in fetuses that are periviable (Figure 12.2—previous page). Additionally, premature infants have less reserve during times of stress (including labor), requiring increased surveillance and vigilance. The premature umbilical cord is thinner with less Wharton's jelly and thus lacks the "cushioning" and structural support of term umbilical cord. Preterm fetuses, therefore, are more prone to umbilical cord compression, which can manifest as large, repetitive, variable decelerations on the FHR tracing during labor. These must be distinguished from the more common, mild-moderate variable decelerations that coincide with normal fetal movement at early gestational ages (Figure 12.2—previous page).

In preterm pregnancies, the uterus is smaller and the fundus is lower in the maternal abdomen than at term. Tocodynamometers and FHR transducers must be placed accordingly for accurate monitoring. Special attention should be paid to tocodynamometer and FHR transducer placement in growth-restricted, preterm fetuses and patients with preterm premature rupture of membranes, as the anatomical differences between these pregnancies and normal term pregnancies can be quite dramatic. The fundus and fetal heart may be below the umbilicus, even in the third trimester. Palpation of the abdomen may facilitate accurate placement of the tocodynamometer and can help to determine whether or not contractions are present. Alternatively, ultrasound may be needed to find the fundus and the fetal heart and hand-holding the monitors may be necessary in order to obtain an accurate and continuous FHR tracing in these particularly challenging preterm patients.

FETAL ANOMALIES

With the exception of growth restriction from uteroplacental insufficiency and certain central nervous system malformations, a fetus with a congenital anomaly will usually have a normal FHR tracing. Fetal circulation is unique in that, even in the presence of most major fetal cardiac anomalies, FHR and fetal oxygenation is normal, resulting in a normal FHR tracing. There are a few notable exceptions, however, wherein the fetal heart's conducting system is altered by structural defects or autoimmune-mediated fibrosis. These fetuses can develop congenital complete heart block, characterized by persistent bradycardia unrelated to oxygenation or fetal compromise (see below).

For the fetus with severe neurologic impairment, either congenital (e.g., anencephaly) or acquired (e.g., in-utero stroke), FHR tracings may show a variety of changes, including "wandering" baselines (due to absent or unstable autonomic function), mild bradycardia, and/or decreased or absent variability due to blunted central sympathetic and parasympathetic signaling (Figure 12.3—next page). These fetuses may have poor responses to vibroacoustic stimulation, as the expected fetal response (stimulation with subsequent movement and acceleration in FHR) is largely under cortical control. Anencephalic fetuses (absent fetal cranium) will often exhibit extreme early decelerations during labor, as the neural tissue is unprotected (Figure 12.4).

156

Figure 12.3: "Wandering" Baseline Seen in an Infant with Absent Brainstem Structures at Term. Umbilical Cord pH Confirmed the Absence of Fetal Acidosis

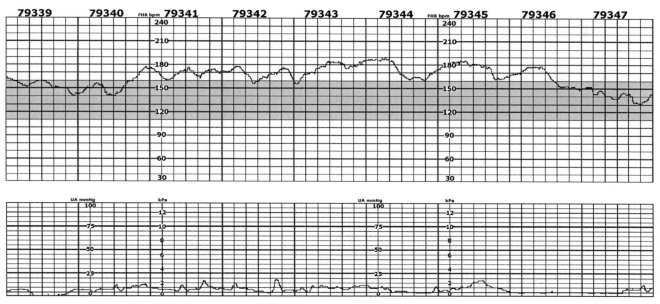

Figure 12.4: Severe Early Decelerations and Minimal Variability in a Fetus with Anencephaly

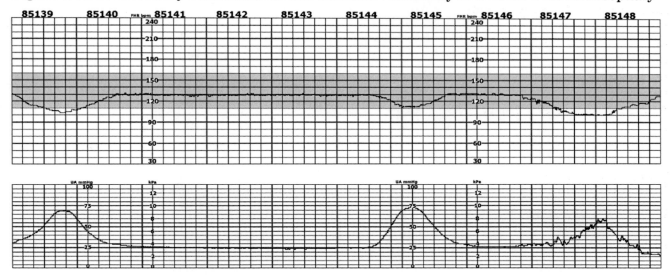

FETAL CARDIAC DEFECTS

As discussed above, fetal cardiac defects are rarely detected by fetal monitoring unless there is an associated arrhythmia. This can be confusing for both patients and providers because the fetal heartbeat "sounds strong and regular," even when there is a severe structural defect. Patients often ask, "How can the provider say that my baby's heart sounds good, but then tell me that its heart isn't normal?" For most affected fetuses, the rhythm of the heart *is* normal, as is the fetal oxygenation status. Therefore, fetal monitoring appears normal as well. For these patients, it is important to help families distinguish between the purpose of FHR monitoring, which assesses fetal oxygenation, and echocardiography, which assesses fetal cardiac structure and function.

While in-utero, oxygen is provided to the fetus by the placenta, rather than the fetal lungs. Normal (postnatal) cardiopulmonary circulation is not required for oxygen delivery before birth. Even when fetal heart structures are abnormal, the unique functions of the fetal ductus venosus and foramen ovale (see also Chapter 3) allow blood from the two sides of the heart to mix, maintaining overall normal fetal oxygen saturation. At birth, however, once the umbilical cord is cut, both of these conduits close, and the lungs are expected to take over for the placenta. It is at that time that abnormal blood flow from congenital cardiac disease can cause serious hypoxemia in the newborn, and the new parents (and the obstetricians) are grateful for the skills and efforts of the neonatologist and pediatric cardiologist. In some cases, prostaglandins will be administered to maintain an open ductus and allow the blood to continue to flow to the lungs.

FETAL CARDIAC ARRHYTHMIAS

In the normal fetal heart, the sinus node in the right atrium initiates and transmits an electrical signal, causing the muscles of the heart to contract. The signal travels through the atrium, traverses the atrioventricular (AV) node, continues down the Purkinje fibers, and ultimately flows to the ventricular walls. Whereas blockage of the pathway at the AV node or Purkinje system can slow the heart, accessory pathways sometimes allow the impulse to cycle back around the AV node and reenter the atrium prematurely. This event can stimulate subsequent atrial contractions, causing a rapid heartbeat (referred to in this context as a tachyarrhythmia, distinct from a secondary tachycardia due to fever or hypoxia). There are a large number of causes of fetal tachy/bradycardias and tachy/bradyarrhythmias (Table 12.1).

Table 12.1: Some Intrinsic Causes of Fetal Arrhythmias

Tachycardias Maternal/Fetal Complications	Bradycardias Maternal/Fetal Complications
➢ Fetal myocarditis (e.g., viral or autoimmune) ➢ Maternal antibodies affecting fetal conduction (e.g., Graves' disease and thyroid-stimulating antibodies)	➢ Fetal hypothyroidism ➢ Fetal hydrops ➢ Fetal CNS anomalies, e.g.: anencephaly/hydrocephaly, fetal stroke
Conditions Resulting in Tachyarrhythmias	**Conditions Resulting in Bradyarrhythmias**
➢ Supraventricular tachycardia (SVT) ➢ Paroxysmal atrial tachycardia (PAT) ➢ Atrial fibrillation or flutter ➢ Premature atrial contractions (PAC) ➢ Premature ventricular contractions (PVC)	➢ Prolonged QT syndrome ➢ Maternal antibodies affecting fetal conduction (Anti-Ro/La) ➢ Structural fetal cardiac disease

As discussed in Chapter 6, the external fetal monitor uses a Doppler ultrasound device that transmits and receives ultrasound signals. The monitor does not "listen" to the beating fetal heart. It instead analyzes patterns and waves of valve movement with Doppler signaling, sampling these waveforms to estimate heart rate. The logic function of an external fetal monitor directs the monitor's microprocessors to reject FHR changes (interval differences) that are excessively different (too slow, too fast) from one another, making the assumption that these are more likely to be due to signaling artifact than physiologic abnormalities. For the fetus with a significant arrhythmia, however, this logic can make external fetal monitoring especially difficult. For the fetus with tachycardia greater than 200 bpm, the logic system, therefore, tends to reject impulses that are "too close" to each other, counting every-other impulse resulting in an FHR tracing that is half the real-life FHR.

For the fetus with a tachy- or brady**arrhythmia** (as opposed to a secondary tachy- or brady**cardia**), marked blunting or absence of variability coupled with a lack of accelerations and decelerations can be expected due to lack of fetal cardiac response to sympathetic and parasympathetic signals. The resultant FHR tracing is therefore less indicative of fetal oxygenation status. As such, when a sustained fetal arrhythmia is present, FHR monitoring is not an accurate measure of fetal well-being. Instead, an alternative method often is used (typically, ultrasound in conjunction with biophysical profile). Monitoring these fetuses during labor is especially difficult in both of these situations given that fetuses with cardiac arrhythmias are predisposed to compromise.

With external monitoring, distinguishing maternal and fetal heart rates can be difficult if they are similar. For example, in a pregnant woman with tachycardia, or in a fetus with bradycardia, the fetal and maternal heart rates may sound the same. Worse, with a demised fetus, the external monitor may measure the maternal pulse, thus providing artificial reassurance. This error can happen even with internal monitoring. Depending on the monitor type, the incoming maternal R-wave signal may be amplified and the maternal heart rate will be detected and counted from the scalp of a deceased or bradycardic fetus. Therefore, assessment of the maternal pulse in these situations is important to confirm that a distinct FHR is being traced.

CONGENITAL BRADYCARDIA

Fetal bradycardia is defined as a sustained heart rate less than 110 beats per minute (bpm) for at least ten minutes. Most acute fetal bradycardia is not due to cardiac structural or conduction abnormalities, but rather to extrinsic factors such as hypoxemia or beta-adrenergic antagonists (see Chapter 6). For these bradycardias, FHR tracings reveal decreased variability and generally do not improve until the extrinsic factor is resolved.

Figure 12.5: Fetal Congenital Heart Block from Heterotaxia Syndrome.
(The fetus received multiple surgeries and pacemakers, but died at three months of life.) Note the lack of variability as well as the bradycardia

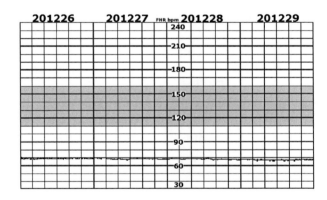

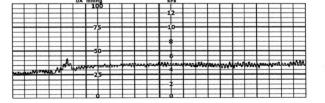

In contrast, hypoxemia rarely is the cause of bradycardia in a fetus with congenital heart disease or a conduction defect. Acquired congenital heart block usually is secondary to transplacental passage of maternal autoantibodies, such as Anti-Ro or Anti-La (also called SSA and SSB). These autoantibodies can attack the fetal cardiac conduction system and result in slow transmissions or disconnections within electrical system of the heart. One particularly dramatic example of such a bradyarrhythmia is complete heart block. In these cases, the atrial and ventricular contractions are completely dissociated from and independent of each other. The sinus node controls the atrial rate and the 55-to-60 bpm ventricular rate reflects a ventricular escape rhythm. The pacer behind this ventricular escape rhythm is inactive as long as the ventricles receive impulses of greater than or equal to 60/min from the atrium. However, the pacer takes control of the ventricle in the absence of atrial signals across the AV node or when atrial signals become too infrequent. This protection prevents the heart from stopping completely. This function is also demonstrated during complete umbilical cord compression, which causes increased parasympathetic tone, obstructing the fetal sinus node and causing FHR decelerations. Because of the protective ventricular pacer, these decelerations rarely go below 50 to 60 bpm.

Congenital bradycardia secondary to structural fetal heart disease is sometimes detectable as early as the first trimester, while autoimmune-mediated complete heart block does not typically present until the second (or more rarely third) trimesters. Most affected fetuses accommodate the slow heart rate surprisingly well, although there is a risk of hydrops fetalis. If bradycardia persists until term, debate invariably ensues regarding mode of delivery, as fetal status cannot be accurately monitored with conventional methods during labor. In these cases, it becomes unclear if and when intervention is indicated because the FHR is no longer a good indicator of fetal hypoxemia. In complete heart block, variability and decelerations will typically be absent because of a lack of vagal (parasympathetic) innervation of the ventricle, although the ventricle may still respond to sympathetic signals (Figure 12.5—previous page).

Rarely, an obstetrician may have the experience of seeing an ostensibly normal pregnant woman for a routine office visit at 30 weeks, and finding the FHR to be 60 bpm. What intervention is indicated? The most obvious response is to call an ambulance and rush the woman to the hospital, not stopping until she reaches the operating room for a stat cesarean section. The most common result of such intervention is delivery of a preterm fetus with normal umbilical cord blood gases and complete heart block for which neonatal cardiac pacing now is considerably more difficult considering the combination of low birth weight and pulmonary immaturity. The mother in these cases often is found to have sub-clinical collagen vascular disease, with positive anti-Ro or La antibodies in the absence of any clinical maternal symptoms. Undiagnosed structural cardiac disease is also a major concern.

What *should* have been done? A bedside ultrasound can be used to confirm that the fetal heart rate is indeed as low as auscultated. Additionally, m-mode evaluation can assess the atrial and ventricular rates independently, discerning whether there is one-to-one conduction or atrioventricular dissociation. In cases of prolonged bradycardia caused by an acute hypoxic event in the office, the inciting catastrophe is unlikely to have occurred before the moment of FHR auscultation. Even if it had occurred just then, by the time the patient was transferred to the hospital and the infant was delivered, the degree of hypoxia—and the associated appearance of the FHR tracing—would likely have been agonal with nearly 100% likelihood of severe neurologic injury or death.

FETAL TACHYARRHYTHMIAS

The majority of tachycardias are not due to fetal cardiac defects, but are instead due to extrinsic factors such as fever, drugs, dehydration, or hypoxia (see Chapter 6). For these tachycardias, FHRs typically are recorded between 160 and 200 bpm and generally will have at least some retained variability. External fetal monitors are capable of recording these rates, and correction of the underlying disorders usually will correct the tachycardia.

However, when heart rates exceed this, there is the possibility that this is instead a tachy**arrhythmia**, not a simple tachy**cardia**, which requires (Table 12.1—page 158), treatment and an understanding of the underlying physiology. For the fetus with supraventricular tachycardia, the FHR will be in excess of 240 bpm, beyond what the logic system of the external FHR monitor can interpret (Figure 12.6—next page). These FHR tracings often will record a rate that is half or one-third that of the real FHR and appears to have minimal variability, since the fetal heart is no longer able to respond to further autonomic influences, and the logic of the external monitor has become overwhelmed. Use of an internal monitor also may be inadequate for monitoring these fetuses because the time between each beat is too brief to allow the monitor to accurately process the information.

The best way to monitor such a fetus is to convert the arrhythmia to a normal rhythm, or suppress it to a more normal range. Depending on the etiology and gestational age at the time of diagnosis of the tachyarrhythmia, some are amenable to in-utero therapy. Formal fetal echocardiography should be able to discern the type of tachycardia (Table 12.1—page 158), and pediatric cardiology should be consulted to help determine optimal medical therapy. Without therapy, sustained tachyarrhythmias can result in fetal circulatory failure, hydrops fetalis, and possible demise. Even partial success in restoring normal sinus rhythm is better than no effort made, because intermittent tachycardia (or lowering the heart rate even if tachycardia persists) is better tolerated by the fetus. This partial success provides much needed periods of a more-normal rate and rhythm, which allow for fetal recovery.

Figure 12.6: Examples of Fetal Tachycardias
(A) Fetal tachycardia secondary to maternal fever and chorioamnionitis
(B) Fetal SVT. The heart rate is visible at the top of the recorded range

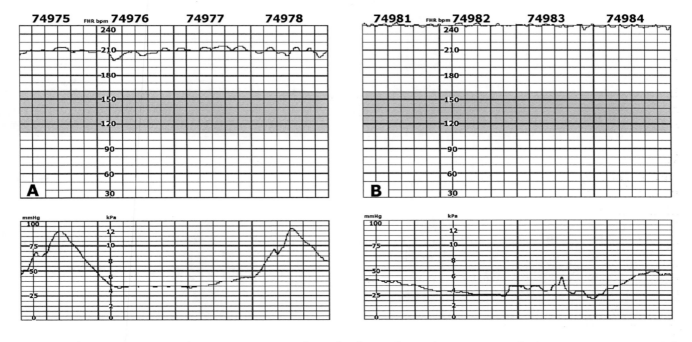

For the fetus in whom there is an irregular rhythm, the most common being premature atrial contractions (PAC—generally from an "ectopic" focus within the right atrium), the resulting FHR tracing is often ascribed to "artifact" or "noise" (Figure 12.7—next page). In cases of PACs, this occurs because the adjacent beats are premature and are followed by a non-compensatory pause to reset the sinus node. There is enough space between beats for the logic system of the monitors to interpret the pattern. The FHR tracing reflects these seemingly erratic changes with an initial spike upwards (the representation of an apparently instantaneous increase in heart rate), followed by a downward spike (the representation of an apparently instantaneous decrease in heart rate), and finally by resumption of the normal rate and rhythm (until the next PAC). Premature atrial contractions are heard on the monitor as irregular beats; sometimes they are isolated, and sometimes they occur in pairs or are heard at every-third-beat (bigeminy or trigeminy). Although they can sound worrisome when frequent, PACs are almost always benign and resolve after birth. The biggest risk is degeneration into a tachyarrhythmia. This is rare, but intermittent antenatal auscultation of the heart rate is recommended. Frequent PACs complicate intrapartum monitoring, but variability, accelerations, and decelerations still will be discernible.

Figure 12.7: Two Examples of Fetal PACs
Note the periodic "noise" or vertical lines within the fetal heart rates. The one on the right is much more severe, which makes monitoring difficult. This generally is a benign finding and resolves after birth.

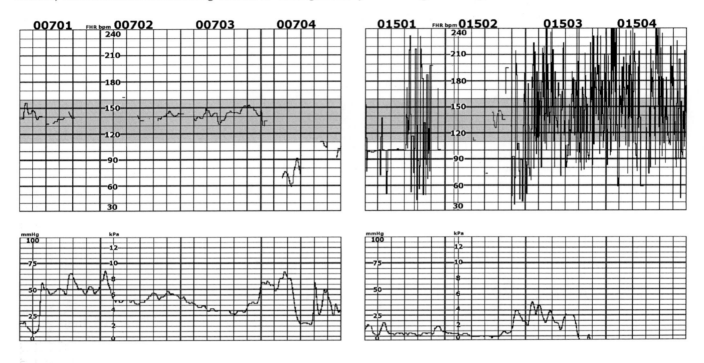

INTRAOPERATIVE FETAL MONITORING

Elective procedures should be avoided during pregnancy; however, surgery sometimes becomes necessary due to deterioration of a known maternal condition, development of a new maternal condition, or for pregnancy-related indications (e.g., cerclage). Ideally, these surgeries should take place in the second trimester when the risks of preterm delivery are lower, but this is not always possible. Assessment of the FHR in surgical patients is necessary.

When the gestational age is pre- or periviable, obtaining a heart rate (Doptone) pre- and post-operatively is sufficient. However, when surgery is performed after the age of viability (greater than or equal to 23 to 24 weeks), some degree of monitoring may need to be considered, depending on the duration and severity of the surgery needed. At minimum, FHR and contraction monitoring before and after the procedure is indicated. Intraoperative monitoring may be considered at and after viability, as long as it is feasible to perform monitoring safely (i.e., it will not compromise the operative field or the maternal outcome), the woman consents to the possibility of emergency cesarean delivery, the appropriate facilities are available to care for any delivered infant, and the nature of the surgical procedure is such that safe interruption for emergency delivery is possible. As always, maternal health concerns outweigh those of the fetus, and any delay of maternal care for transfer or arranging fetal monitoring that would be detrimental to maternal health or outcome should be avoided.

It is best to optimize circumstances preoperatively, rather than react to abnormalities intraoperatively. The patient should be properly positioned with care taken to avoid supine

162

hypotensive syndrome. This will minimize positional and hypotension-related FHR changes and may prevent intraoperative intervention for preventable FHR tracing abnormalities. Cardiopulmonary optimization may include lateral tilt (if possible, even to a small degree) to minimize vena cava compression, as well as oxygen supplementation and fluid resuscitation prior to induction of general anesthesia with the goal of avoiding hypoxia and hypotension. Good communication between the surgical and obstetric teams is vital to good patient outcomes.

Although there are no known teratogenic effects for standard doses of anesthetic agents, sedation and inhalational agents given to the pregnant woman, these will also affect the fetus, leading to decreased fetal movement, loss of accelerations, and decreased variability. Therefore, if continuous fetal monitoring is employed intraoperatively, interpretation is based primarily on the absence of prolonged and persistent decelerations, rather than maintenance of reactivity or a Category I FHR tracing for the entire surgery, which generally will not be present.

Figure 12.8: FHR Tracing Before (A), During (B), and After (C) Electroconvulsive Therapy (ECT)
Note the lack of variability during the procedure, with prompt return after reversal of the anesthetic effects.

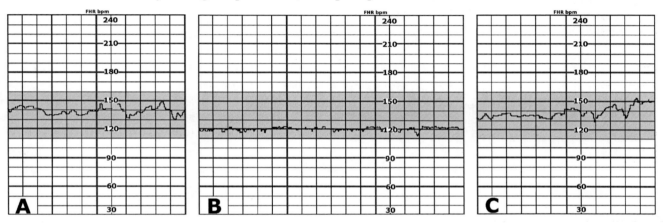

For intraoperative monitoring, ACOG recommends that: "The decision to use fetal monitoring should be individualized and, if used, should be based on gestational age, type of surgery, and facilities available. Ultimately, each case warrants a team approach (anesthesia and obstetric care providers, surgeons, pediatricians, and nurses) for optimal safety of the woman and the fetus."

THE MEDICALLY COMPROMISED PATIENT

Often, those patients with medical complications are also those in whom fetal monitoring is the most critical. In these patients, it is especially important for the provider to understand and react to the physiology specific to the patient's medical diagnoses, and not just to the FHR monitor tracing. When maternal physiology is altered due to medical complications, the fetus is often affected as well. In order to correct FHR tracing abnormalities, the underlying maternal physiology must be considered.

A variety of maternal diseases can result in suboptimal fetal status, especially if the mother is significantly hypoxic or acidotic. The fetus relies on chemical gradients to exchange oxygen, carbon dioxide, and nutrients across the placenta. For this reason, fetal oxygenation is compromised in the setting of maternal hypoxia. When there is maternal hypercarbia (retention of CO_2), the fetus retains CO_2. If there is maternal acidosis, fetal pH will fall as well. The FHR tracing may reflect these changes, revealing decreased or absent variability, absent accelerations, and/or late decelerations. For the majority of these situations, compromise is transient and improvement of the maternal condition will result in improvement of fetal status and subsequent normalization of the FHR tracing. The provider caring for a profoundly ill pregnant woman must be aware of the additional stress associated with delivery for both the woman and the fetus. This additional stress may cause further deterioration of an already compromised patient, and may add to the challenges faced by a premature infant with pre-existing acidemia. Therefore, in order to improve an abnormal FHR tracing, the provider should focus on correcting or optimizing the underlying maternal condition. If the maternal condition is rapidly reversible, treatment may save an unnecessary premature delivery. In cases when maternal condition further deteriorates and Category III FHR tracings persist, decisions regarding delivery require multidisciplinary input from the patient or patient family, the obstetrician, pediatrician, and the medical/surgical teams caring for the pregnant woman.

Figure 12.9: Category III FHR Tracing
A woman with respiratory compromise and severe acidosis from status asthmaticus; the fetus returned to a Category I FHR tracing with correction of the maternal condition.

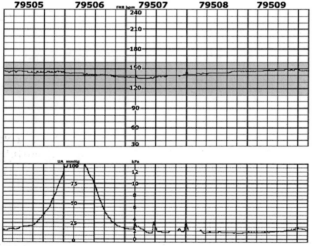

A pertinent example of the impact that maternal condition can have on FHR tracing is the mother with diabetic ketoacidosis (DKA). This occurs when a lack of insulin leads to severe metabolic derangement. In this complication, maternal acidosis (pH less than 7.3, and in extreme cases, pH less than 7.0) occurs secondary to accumulation of organic ketoacids, namely β-hydroxybutyrate and acetoacetate. This buildup of ketoacids results in a compensatory decrease in serum HCO_3^- (bicarbonate) concentration, generally to less than 10 mEq/L. Ketoacidosis causes dehydration, electrolyte abnormalities, impaired placental perfusion, and fetal acidosis from placental transfer of maternal ketoacids, all of which lead to ominous FHR patterns that, under usual circumstances, would mandate delivery (Figure 12.9). However, these Category III FHR abnormalities will rapidly resolve with appropriate treatment of maternal DKA. Thus, delivery should not be undertaken until the woman has been stabilized, treated, and the subsequent fetal response has been evaluated. Delivery prior to stabilization of the mother can result in worsening of DKA, further metabolic derangement, and subsequent maternal neurologic injury or death.

CONCLUSION

Although FHR monitoring is an important tool in assessing fetal status, there are special circumstances that may limit its application and interpretation. In some cases, standard monitoring routines can be modified to achieve success. At other times, the treatment of underlying disorders should precede intervention for abnormalities in FHR tracing.

RELATED READINGS

1. American College of Obstetricians and Gynecologists (2011). Nonobstetric surgery during pregnancy. ACOG Practice Bulletin #474.

2. Benova L, Mohamoud YA, Calvert C, and Abu-Raddad LJ (2014). Vertical transmission of hepatitis C virus: Systematic review and meta-analysis. Clinical Infectious Diseases, 69(6): 765-773

3. Carroll MA and Yeomans ER (2005). Diabetic ketoacidosis in pregnancy. Critical Care Medicine, 33(10): S347-S353.

4. Duff P, Sweet RL, and Edwards RK (2009). Maternal and fetal infections (Chapter 38). IN: RK Creasy, R Resnik, JD Iams, Lockwood CJ, Moore TR (Eds.) Creasy and Resnik's Maternal-Fetal Medicine: Principles and Practice (Ed. 6), Philadelphia, PA: W.B. Saunders Company, pp. 739-795.

5. Krebs H, Petres R, Dunn L, et al. (1979). FHR monitoring I. Classification and prognosis of FHR patterns. American Journal of Obstetrics and Gynecology, 133:762-772.

6. Glantz JC and Bertoia N (2011). Preterm nonstress testing: 10-beat compared with 15-beat criteria. Obstetrics and Gynecology, 118(1):87-93.

7. Krebs H, Petres R, Dunn L, Jordaan HV, and Segreti A (1979). Intrapartum fetal heart rate monitoring I. Classification and prognosis of fetal heart rate patterns. American Journal of Obstetrics and Gynecology, 133:762-772.

8. Nageotte MP and Gilstrap LC (2009). Intrapartum fetal surveillance (Chapter 22). IN: RK Creasy, R Resnik, JD Iams, Lockwood CJ, Moore TR (Eds.) Creasy and Resnik's Maternal-Fetal Medicine: Principles and Practice (Ed. 6), Philadelphia, PA: W.B. Saunders Company, pp. 400-405.

9. Park Y, Park S, Kim Y, Hoh J, Park Y, and Park M (2010). Computerized fetal heart rate monitoring after vibroacoustic stimulation in the anencephalic fetus. Early Human Development, 86(9):569-572.

10. Peleg D and Goldman JA (1979). Fetal heart patterns: A study of the anencephalic fetus. Obstetrics and Gynecology, 53(4):530-533.

11. Thornburg L (2011). Antepartum obstetrical complications associated with obesity. Seminars in Perinatology, 35:317-323.

Chapter 12 Review
Fetal Monitoring in the Complex Patient

1. Internal fetal heart rate monitoring (FSE) is to be avoided in patients with:

    A. prior, resolved hepatitis B infection.
    B. group B *Streptococcus*.
    C. human immunodeficiency virus disease.
    D. active tuberculosis.

2. Strategies for improved monitoring in the severely obese patient include:

    A. cesarean section to avoid monitoring all together.
    B. laying the patient flat.
    C. using multiple monitor belts tied together so they encircle the patient's abdomen.
    D. using pillows and rolls to angle the FHR transducer and secure the tocodynamometer .

3. True or False. When performing a nonstress test on a patient with a gestational age of 30 weeks, you note that there are accelerations that meet the criteria for reactivity in fetuses less than 32 weeks' gestation. In addition, you note several variable decelerations. You know that there is an increased risk for variable decelerations in a preterm infant because the umbilical cord is thin and lacks Wharton's jelly.

    A. True
    B. False

4. For the fetus with a cardiac defect, the fetal heart rate will sound regular in rhythm and rate. This is because:

    A. oxygen delivery for the fetus occurs at the placenta level.
    B. the foramen ovale and ductus arteriosus allow for the mixing of blood from both sides of the heart to maintain normal fetal oxygenation.
    C. the muscular structure of the umbilical arteries ensures the unhindered transport of oxygenated blood to the fetus.
    D. structural anomalies of the fetal heart generally will not affect the rhythm or rate during fetal monitoring unless there also is a conduction disorder or arrhythmia.
    E. All of the above.
    F. A and B only.
    G. B and C only.

5. When complete heart block occurs in the fetus, the heart rate auscultated is the ventricular rate. The range for the ventricular rate in the fetus is:

    A. 55 to 60 bpm.
    B. 65 to 70 bpm.
    C. 75 to 80 bpm.

Chapter 12 Review Answers
Fetal Monitoring in the Complex Patient

1. **The correct answer is C.** It is plausible that any break in the fetal skin would provide access for the virus, resulting in the fetus/neonate becoming infected.

2. **The correct answer is D.** Performing a cesarean section for obesity alone only would increase the patient's morbidity. Laying the patient flat will result in supine hypotension and decrease uteroplacental blood flow. By tying multiple belts together, pressure points may occur and result in skin breakdown.

3. **The correct answer is A.** Wharton's jelly (the thick, jelly portion of the umbilical cord) protects the umbilical cord from compression and usually doesn't appear until the latter part of the third trimester.

4. **The correct answer is D.** A and B are true but do not affect the "sound" of the fetal heart beat during fetal heart rate monitoring.

5. **The correct answer is A.**

Chapter 13

Patient Safety and Team Communication: Developing a Culture of Safety and Teamwork

INTRODUCTION

The past decade has seen a proliferation in research and analysis of patient safety and teamwork in healthcare. Despite these efforts, a comprehensive model of team performance specific to medical settings has not been fully developed. Rather, medicine has utilized and built on successful team models from aviation, nuclear power, and military science. The current approaches to patient safety and teamwork in healthcare in general and obstetrics in particular are reviewed below.

SOURCES OF ERROR

One of the principle findings of the Institute of Medicine (IOM) report *"To Err Is Human: Building a Safer Health System"* was that systemic failures in the delivery of healthcare account for more errors than does poor performance by individuals. Because systemic successes and failures depend to a great extent on the performance of teams, the report recommended interdisciplinary team training to reduce the incidence of medical errors.

As the federal leader in implementing the IOM recommendations, the Agency for Healthcare Research and Quality (AHRQ) established the High Reliability Organizations (HRO) Network and developed Team Strategies and Tools to Enhance Performance and Patient Safety (TeamSTEPPS). Through extensive review of human factors, teamwork, and Crew Resource Management (CRM) research, critical components of HRO and teamwork have been identified and incorporated into TeamSTEPPS for use in healthcare settings.

TEAMS AND THEIR ROLE IN PATIENT SAFETY

By definition, teams are comprised of a group of individuals with shared willingness to cooperate towards a common mission or goal. In healthcare, high functioning teams can be identified as having interrelated knowledge, skills, and attitudes (KSA). Additionally, these teams have the ability to adapt to the needs and actions of others as well as a shared understanding about the specific procedures being performed and/or the patient population cared for. Teams in the perinatal setting are dynamic, while the common KSA and shared mission remain static. The core areas of the AHRQ's TeamSTEPPS program include development of team leadership, situation monitoring, mutual support, and communication (Table 13.1). These were developed to meet the needs of healthcare organizations and provide a road map for promoting a stronger culture of patient safety and quality care.

Table 13.1: TeamSTEPPS Program
Team strategies and tools to enhance performance and develop a culture of patient safety

Team leadership	Develops the abilities of leadership to direct and coordinate activities of team members. • Assess team performance • Assign tasks • Develop team knowledge and skills • Motivate team members • Plan and organize • Establish a positive team atmosphere.
Situation monitoring	• Capacity to develop common understandings of the team environment • Apply appropriate strategies to monitor teammate performance accurately
Mutual support	• Anticipate other team members' needs and shift workload among members to achieve balance
Communication	• Develop an efficient exchange of information • Consult with other team members, including the patient

Obviously, there are a great many factors that may impede successful perinatal team development (Table 13.2). As a result, developing a culture that supports perinatal teamwork often takes years of progressive initiatives. Building on easy wins towards more complex problem solving can help maintain a positive focus. Often, regression to previous patterns of interacting will occur before lasting change is established. Continual redirection and leadership support toward the common mission of patient-safety-centered care may be required. Commitment to change needs to be reinforced by facilitating bi-directional sharing of information between leadership and frontline staff. Ultimately, in the face of increasing fiscal and regulatory pressure to improve service, safety, and quality of healthcare, the resulting advantages of team-based care will lead to better patient outcomes and healthier organizations.

Table 13.2: Some Barriers to Successful Team Building

> ➢ Historic role of women in society
> ➢ Traditional roles of physicians and nurses
> ➢ Institutional territory and politics
> ➢ Differences in licensure
> ➢ Differences in professional accountability
> ➢ Type and quantity of education
> ➢ Different styles of learning
> ➢ Different styles of information exchange
> ➢ Methods and amounts of compensation
> ➢ Social and professional positions
> ➢ Unresolved prior conflicts
> ➢ Lack of common incentives

HUMAN FACTORS ENGINEERING

Human Factors Engineering (HFE) is a discipline that involves the application of what is known about human capabilities and limitations to the design of products, processes, systems, and work environments. Its applicability to error in healthcare is just beginning to be appreciated. Human Factors Engineering can be applied to the design of all systems having a human interface, and its application improves ease of use, system performance and reliability, and user satisfaction, while reducing operational errors, operator stress, training requirements, user fatigue, and, ultimately, liability. Because human factors arguably are the key to development of a culture of safety, studies of the interactions between humans and technology are crucial to understanding the individual and environmental factors that can lead to medical error.

One example of HFE is the impact of the human factor on interpretation of electronic fetal monitoring (EFM). Visit most modern labor and delivery units and there will be an array of screens displaying the fetal heart rate (FHR) tracings to assure that the team responds in a timely manner to any Category II or III FHR tracing. However, recent work suggests that as the number of EFM displays increased, participants detected fewer critical signals (i.e., late FHR decelerations). Additionally, as time on the task (watching EFM screens) increased, the ability to detect critical signals (i.e., late FHR decelerations) decreased. This underlies the need for a team approach to vigilance and rotating task assignment to minimize the negative impact of losing situational awareness due to fatigue, stress, and workload.

TEAM COMMUNICATION

Importance of Team Communication in EFM

A report of sentinel events for all areas of medicine in 2006 by the Joint Commission indicated that communication failures among professionals caused the vast majority (70%) of reported events, with a very high mortality in these events (75%). For those involved in perinatal care, professional liability and patient harm involves three main areas of clinical risk: EFM, induction/augmentation of labor, and second-stage labor management. Team communication is a core skill crucial to the use and interpretation of EFM, and the management of labor and delivery.

EFM and Team Communication

Keeping in mind the team concepts of shared KSA (Knowledge, Skills, and Attitude), consideration should be given to recommending that all care providers learn EFM in a similar way and have ongoing professional development in this area. Elevating the education of the perinatal team in this critical area of knowledge can be accomplished through interdisciplinary training of the skills involved in the technical aspects of equipment use, assessment of FHR and uterine contraction pattern, and decision-making algorithms related to FHR interpretation. Interdisciplinary training sessions also can provide opportunities for team building and consistency in base knowledge. Continuing support for open dialogue and sharing knowledge surrounding EFM interpretation can be accomplished by providing routine opportunities for interdisciplinary case and strip review/discussion sessions and allow staff to practice effective conflict resolution skills. These sessions should be conducted in an open, respectful forum that allows for equal contribution to practice and decision-making discussions.

The three key elements to affect team communication are:

1. use of common terminology,
2. an organized structure, and
3. timely and accurate documentation.

Sharing a Common Terminology

An important element of effective communication of EFM interpretation is that all care providers share a common language for interpretation. Utilizing the NICHD terminology to describe FHR patterns assures a common language as the basis for communication and documentation of FHR interpretation for the perinatal team.

Table 13.3: Tools for Organizing Communication

Tool/Strategy	Definition and Use
SBAR (Situation, Background, Assessment, Recommendation/Request)	Communication of important information during routine updates and transitions of care, including exchange of critical information requiring immediate attention/action
Call-Out	Used in situations where it is necessary to simultaneously inform all team members present of important information (such as during a prolonged FHR deceleration)
Check Back	Ensure that information conveyed is understood as intended. Closes the loop on information exchanged. *Example*: Physician: "Please give the patient terbutaline, and I will be there in five minutes." RN: "I am giving terbutaline 0.25 mg subcutaneously one time for tachysystole. You will be here to evaluate the patient in five minutes."

Communication at Transitions of Care

Efficient communication also requires an organized structure to relay information effectively between individuals during routine updates, especially when the information requires either notification of changes in FHR patterns or transitions in care. TeamSTEPPS provides multiple examples of tools helpful for the organization of information which include: SBAR (Situation, Background, Assessment, Recommendation/Request); Call out (generally used during urgent situations); and Check Back (Table 13.3)

Handoffs—Importance of Standardized Approach

Handoffs are moments in the course of patient care that are particularly vulnerable to information misinterpretations and omissions. Utilizing a standardized handoff method, such as SBAR (Table 13.3), in handoffs gives an organization strategy to help assure that information for critical analysis of FHR monitoring is provided. However, at a minimum, handoffs should include the maternal and fetal condition during the prior shift, as well as any FHR changes and the team responses (Table 13.4).

Handoffs also provide an opportunity to jointly review the historic FHR tracing, which is an ideal way to assure that periodic changes are noted (i.e., a rise in baseline over 12 hours may be unnoticed if only the prior one to two hours of the FHR are reviewed). Development of paper or electronic tools that include FHR assessments are helpful in promoting a tangible handoff that optimizes efficient and effective information exchange for nurse-to-nurse and nurse-to-physician communication.

Table 13.4: Minimum Required Information for Handoffs

> - Course of labor progress (if laboring)
>
> - Maternal condition and medical concerns
>
> - Category of FHR over the past shift including:
>   - Uterine contraction pattern and interventions
>   - Baseline and variability
>   - Presence or absence of accelerations
>   - Presence or absence, type, timeframe and clinical context of any decelerations
>
> - Actions taken and fetal response to intrauterine resuscitation
>
> - Recommendations and follow-up considerations

Bedside Reporting at Handoff

Recently, the practice of bedside report during nurse-to-nurse change of shift has become incorporated into standard practice for many perinatal inpatient settings. Bedside handoff allows an opportunity for the patient to participate in the information exchange and can promote building a trusting, open and safe environment for both the clinicians and patient/family. In one study, the higher that women as patients rated the amount and quality of the information about EFM provided by the nurse during initial monitor application, the more positively they viewed their overall experience during labor. In addition, women who felt that they were adequately informed about interventions during episodes of Category II and III FHR patterns were less likely to become overly concerned and anxious.

Handoff Communication—Value of Team Approach

Incorporating interdisciplinary team activities into the handoff procedure also can help to minimize the potential for lapses in information. These can include briefings, team huddles, and debriefings as part of routine practice. They also provide an opportunity for team collaboration and consensus about FHR interpretation and plan-of-care decisions. Building a practice of routine one- to two-minute debriefing discussions during handoffs, discussions that include all appropriate, immediately involved members of the team (nurse, resident staff, providers, anesthesia staff, pediatrics, etc.), allows for exchange of information between providers. This is important, especially if a procedure or intervention is planned or ongoing, or if the fetus or mother is critically ill. Additionally, it assures that all care providers are aware of the critical information in the situation, that their concerns have been addressed, and that there is a consensus on the plan moving forward.

DOCUMENTATION

The final and arguably one of the most important aspects of communication is appropriate documentation. It is a critical part of effective, efficient, and timely communication. The medical record, be it paper or electronic, tells the story of the patient's clinical course and interface with the healthcare environment. The medical record not only provides a mode of communication between care providers, it also provides support for financial reimbursement of care, and allows for quality assurance, utilization review, and regulatory audits. The medical record often is the primary exhibit in legal proceedings such as litigation of malpractices suits, family court, social security/disability hearings, and criminal proceedings. The contents of the medical record will be used to support/refute a care provider's testimony and provides written documentation of the team's communication and decision-making process concerning a patient's course of care. The medical record provides validity for decision making and objective evidence of a patient's medical course, determines the chain of command utilized, and documents the communication between consulting services. Memories fade, but documentation remains.

Keys to Appropriate Documentation

Documentation that is consistent, objective, and accurate (COA) should be the goal (Table 13.5). These concepts may seem intuitive, but there are many instances of inappropriate use of the medical record for personal commentary (e.g., the word "huh?" with an arrow pointing to another provider's entry) or blaming comments (e.g., "...urgent procedure on hold because anesthesia is poorly staffed...;" "provider yelled at me and hung up during conversation so no orders for treating tachysystole obtained."). While in and of themselves not the cause of a poor outcome or error, inappropriate entries can be used as fodder for a plaintiff attorney or regulatory agency to paint a

Table 13.5: Keys to Documentation

Consistent: Meets the standards set by policy, regulatory requirement, and standards of practice

Objective: State the facts including the situation, background, assessment, and recommendations; free from personal bias, emotion, or subjective statements

Accurate: Date and time, specific details; use of NICHD terminology

less-than-complimentary picture of the care provided to the patient. Documentation that shows failure to utilize the chain of command in the face of concerning FHR patterns also can point to system and institutional failures in the eyes of a jury or regulatory board. An example of this is multiple entries of "MD paged regarding late FHR decelerations with no response" documented over the course of hours. Although perhaps accurate, these statements depict a disregard/lack of institutional support for escalating concerns up a chain of command and, ultimately, will be viewed as a lapse in writing care provider's judgment and patient advocacy. Inconsistencies in the documentation of an FHR event also can create a red flag. Building a practice of routine one- to two-minute debriefing discussions after a situation has stabilized to exchange information between providers following procedures or interventions can enhance consistency of documentation in these circumstances, as well as assure that concerns have been addressed and there is a consistent plan moving forward.

COMMUNICATION CHALLENGES

Developing interdisciplinary teams to discuss and develop consensus in areas prone to conflict in FHR monitoring can provide an opportunity to build team trust as well as minimize conflict in the clinical practice environment. Communication in times of critical, time-sensitive interventions such as those for tachysystole, intrauterine resuscitation, and triggering the chain of command particularly are prone to breakdown. Intrapersonal communication barriers such as professional deference and passive-aggressive behaviors are examples of conflict avoidance strategies that subtly can undermine honest, direct, and timely communication. The tools for effective communication during times of conflict are not commonly taught during most medical professional training but are a crucial skill for all care providers. Therefore, a systematic, team approach is necessary for effective communication among care providers (Table 13.6). TeamSTEPPS provides multiple simple, easy to remember strategies including the "two-challenge rule," "CUS" words (Concerned, Uncomfortable, Safety issue), and the DESC Script. Obviously, before any of these are implemented, the entire team should discuss and drill on strategies related to team building and developing a culture of safety.

Team Communication—The Two-Challenge Rule

For the two-challenge rule, the care provider expresses concerns, advocating and asserting his or her concerns at least twice. In this way, the concerned provider assures that the team receives the information at least twice if the initial assertion is ignored (thus, the name, "two-challenge rule"). These two attempts may come from the same person or two different team members. Ideally, the first challenge should be in the form of a question, thus requiring a response by the other team member. The second challenge should provide some support for the concern (i.e., "I am concerned about this FHR tracing because of the repetitive late decelerations."). The "two-challenge" tactic ensures that an expressed concern has been heard, understood, and acknowledged.

There may be times when an initial assertion is ignored. If after two attempts the concern still is disregarded, but the member believes patient or staff safety is or may be severely compromised, the two-challenge rule mandates that the provider take a stronger course of action using a supervisor or the chain of command. This overcomes the natural tendency to believe the medical team leader must always know what he or she is doing, even when the actions taken depart from established guidelines. When invoking this rule and moving up the chain, it is essential to communicate to the entire medical team that additional input has been solicited.

CUS Words in the Workplace

The idea behind CUS words is that there are specific trigger terms that prompt a response from care providers by using words that suggest the need for an immediate response. The CUS words are such signals, just like the words "critical" and "STAT," because they carry special meaning in the medical community. CUS words and other signal phrases are most effective in spoken communication. When they are used, the team should understand clearly (if appropriately trained on communication as part of ongoing team safety and advocacy measures) that there is not only an issue but also the magnitude of the concern. When a team member encounters a concerning situation, she should use the words, in order, to state and re-state her concerns. The team member states her concern (C), and if these are not addressed, states that she is uncomfortable (U) with continuing. If the situation continues, the member states that this is a safety issue (S). This is synonymous with "stop" and the team must address the situation before care can continue. Ideally, a provider using "CUS" words should state her concern, state a reason for her discomfort and then, if it continues, state that if not resolved it represents an ongoing safety issue. She should be prepared to have a calm, reasoned discussion about the ways that her concern is related to safety, and, also, she should be ready to utilize the chain of command if her concerns are not addressed or acknowledged.

The "DESC" Script

The DESC Script (Describe, Express, Suggest, Consequences) is a methodology of team communication that can be practiced during simulations or drills and utilized to efficiently provide important information and minimize conflict. Although this can be used in any situation, it is best used when resolving personal conflicts such as ongoing patterns of difficult behaviors (hostile, harassing, etc.), or persistent patient safety concerns. The person initiating the discussion (generally as part of a team approach) should describe the specific situation, express his or her concerns regarding the actions or events, suggest alternatives, and state the potential consequences of the situation. The team should reach a consensus on these prior to completing the DESC Script to assure that there is a unified front when approaching the situation. This type of conflict resolution can be time consuming and is best utilized in a non-critical situation.

The discussion should be timed, should occur in a non-public forum, and should focus on *what*, not *who* is right in the situation. The team should reach a win-win situation, and it should be emphasized that blame is not being assigned and that critique is not criticism.

Chain of Command

Inherent in any patient safety program is the development of guidelines and policies for invoking a chain of command when appropriate. Decisive action is needed in times of conflict or disagreement, and therefore, a chain of command is recommended for all perinatal units. The guideline should be simple and straightforward so that all care providers are clear regarding who and how to escalate an immediate patient safety concern. Figure 13.1 outlines an example of a theoretical chain of command for a nurse identifying a patient safety concern. Additionally,

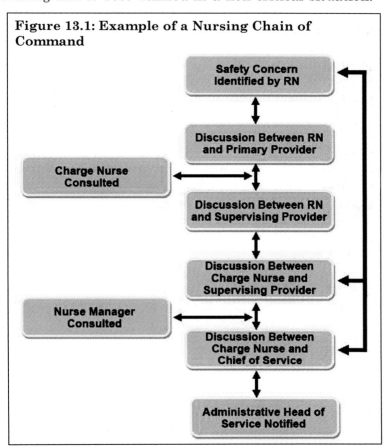

Figure 13.1: Example of a Nursing Chain of Command

Safety Concern Identified by RN

Discussion Between RN and Primary Provider

Charge Nurse Consulted

Discussion Between RN and Supervising Provider

Discussion Between Charge Nurse and Supervising Provider

Nurse Manager Consulted

Discussion Between Charge Nurse and Chief of Service

Administrative Head of Service Notified

many perinatal units have open access to in-house Rapid Response Teams that may be contacted at any point by any member of the care team or patient/patient's family. A clear and direct guideline must be accompanied by a non-punitive response and leadership support for staff when the system is invoked. Administrative response should include validation to the staff involved during debriefing for identifying any potential ongoing or systemic safety issue once the urgent situation is resolved.

Patient and Care Provider Communication Challenges

The unfortunate truth is that most providers practicing obstetrics will be subjected to a lawsuit at least once in their career, with an average of almost three. Two strategies to mitigate this risk include partnering with patients and clearly documenting the course of that partnership. It cannot be emphasized enough that one of the best defenses is consistent, objective, and accurate (COA) documentation of all educational assessments and information provided surrounding the options for care. This is crucial, especially in the context of the patient who makes choices that typically would be considered against medical advice.

In the context of obstetric care, patient autonomy creates the basis for providing enough information for a competent person to make the best decisions for himself or herself and the situation regarding his or her care and treatment. In the daily practice of obstetrics, there are many ethical issues relating to fetal-maternal conflict. When a woman is pregnant, she is expected to present herself to the healthcare provider. Urine and blood samples are expected to be taken. The consent and informed choice to undergo these tests often is taken for granted (educational pamphlets and reading material notwithstanding). When a patient makes a different choice of management, this can create conflict within the perinatal team. Additionally, an ethical dilemma exists when a competent patient and partner make choices that have a potential for poor outcomes for either themselves or their unborn fetus. One of these choices is selection of the mode of intrapartum fetal monitoring. It behooves the perinatal unit to have clear, agreed upon guidelines based on national recommendations for the use of continuous and intermittent monitoring as it relates to high- and low-risk populations, and that these guidelines be shared with patients as part of their pre-admission education. Additionally, providers and patients must be able to have an honest, open, and non-confrontational dialogue about the goals of care, the patient's understanding of alternatives, and the potential consequences of each decision.

CONCLUSION

Safety surrounding FHR monitoring practices involves a distinct set of individual and team skills, knowledge, and attitudes. The perinatal unit can facilitate the development of those particular to FHR monitoring, interpretation, and clinical decision making through a comprehensive strategy embraced by all members of the healthcare team. This must incorporate interdisciplinary education, team training strategies, communication techniques, and conflict management. Guidelines and policies that are developed by interdisciplinary consensus, as well as national best practice guidelines and local regulatory requirements, likely will lead to improved perinatal safety.

ADDITIONAL RESOURCES

Agency for Healthcare Research and Quality: http://www.ahrq.gov/teamsteppstools/

National Patient Safety Foundation: http://www.npsf.org/

Association of Women's Health, Obstetric and Neonatal Nurses: http://www.awhonn.org

American Congress of Obstetricians and Gynecologists: http://www.acog.org/

National Institute of Child Health and Human Development: http://www.nichd.nih.gov/

U.S. Department of Defense Patient Safety Program: http://health.mil/dodpatientsafety.aspx

American Society for Healthcare Risk Management: http://www.ashrm.org/

RELATED READINGS

1.   Analysis of the Current Medical Liability Climate in NYS (ACOG, District II/NY, June 2008)

2.   Anderson BL, Scerbo MW, Belfore LA, and Abuhamad AZ (2011). Time and number of displays impact critical signal detection in fetal heart rate tracings. American Journal of Perinatology, 28(6):435-441.

3.   Baker DP, Day R, and Salas E (2006). Teamwork as an essential component of high-reliability organizations. HSR: Health Services Research, 41:4, Part II, 1576-1595.

4.   Block M, Ehrenworth JF, Cruce VM, Ng'ang'a N, Weinbach J, Saber SB, Milic M, Urgo JA, Sokoli D, and Schlesinger MD (2010). The tangible handoff: A team approach for advancing structured communication in labor and delivery. The Joint Commission Journal on Quality and Patient Safety, 36(6): 282-288.

5.   Clancy CM and Tornberg DN (2007). TeamSTEPPS: Assuring optimal teamwork in clinical settings. American Journal of Medical Quality, 22(3):214-217.

6.   Patterson K, Grenny J, McMillan R, and Switzler A (2002). Move to action: How to turn crucial conversations into action and results (Chapter 9). IN: Crucial Conversations: Tools for Talking When the Stakes are High. New York, NY: McGraw-Hill, pp. 161-178

7.   Schmalenberg K (2009). Nurse-physician relationships in hospitals: 20,000 nurses tell their story. Critical Care Nurse, 29(1):74-83.

8.   Simpson K (2009). Communication of fetal heart monitoring Information (Chapter 8). IN: Fetal Heart Monitoring: Principles and Practices (Ed. 4). Malden: AWHONN, pp. 177-208.

9.   Simpson K (2006). Essential criteria to promote safe care during labor and birth. AWHONN Lifelines, 9(6):478-483.

10.   Simpson KR and Knox GE (2001). Turning rhetoric into reality: Perinatal teamwork. AWHONN Lifelines, 5(5):56-59.

11.   Sirota T (2007). Nurse/physician relationships: Improving or not? Nursing, (37)1:52-55.

12.   TeamSTEPPS™: Strategies & Tools to Enhance Performance and Patient Safety. AHRQ, November, 2008. www.ahrq.gov.

13.   Yeo GS and Lim ML (2011). Maternal and fetal best interests in day-to-day obstetrics. Annals of the Academy of Medicine, Singapore, 40(1):43-47.

Chapter 13 Review

Patient Safety and Team Communication: Developing a Culture of Safety and Teamwork

1. Team training can help to improve:

    A. team leadership.
    B. situation monitoring.
    C. mutual support among teams.
    D. communication.
    E. all of the above.

2. Team leadership skills that enhance performance include:

    A. assessing team performance.
    B. assigning tasks.
    C. assigning blame within teams.
    D. motivating team members.
    E. all of the above.
    F. A, B, and D only.

3. Barriers to creation of successful teams include:

    A. traditional roles.
    B. styles of information exchange.
    C. prior conflicts.
    D. lack of common incentives.
    E. all of the above.

4. Team communications is maximized by:

    A. changing teams to include only people that get along.
    B. support for only a few key members sharing their opinions in a crisis.
    C. using common terminology within teams.
    D. avoiding an organized structure for communication to allow individual style.
    E. saving all documentation until after the end of the shift.

5. Strategies for team communications include:

    A. SBAR: Situation, Background, Assessment, Recommendation/Request.
    B. Call-in: Staff call in and review the team's work over the last shift.
    C. Check-in: Random visits to the unit by leadership.

Chapter 13 Review Answers
Patient Safety and Team Communication:
Developing a Culture of Safety and Teamwork

1. **The correct answer is E.**

2. **The correct answer is F.**

3. **The correct answer is E.**

4. **The correct answer is C.** This is an important element for effective communication in fetal monitor interpretation. Use of NICHD terminology assures a common language as the basis for communication and documentation.

5. **The correct answer is A.** SBAR assures communication of important information during routine updates and transitions of care. Call-in and Check-in are not terms utilized in team training.

Chapter 14

Basic Fetal Heart Rate Interpretation

Clinical Case Study 14.1

F.N. is a 21-year-old, G1 P0000 woman at 40 2/7 weeks' gestation who presents to your labor and delivery unit with a complaint of painful uterine contractions. They started as menstrual-type cramps at approximately 0650 hours this morning. F.N. reports that her fetus is active. She denies loss of fluid and vaginal bleeding.

F.N.'s current pregnancy has been uncomplicated.

F.N.'s past medical history includes seasonal allergies and gastroesophageal reflux disease (GERD). F.N.'s daily medications include a prenatal vitamin; famotidine, 40 mg; and cetirizine, 10 mg. All prenatal testing has been normal, including negative group B *Streptococcus* testing.

The estimated weight of F.N.'s fetus is 3,200 gm.

On admission, F.N.'s cervix is 3 cm dilated, 100% effaced, and the fetal vertex is at -2 station.

F.N.'s admission vital signs are: blood pressure 120/69 mmHg, pulse 74 bpm, respirations 16 rpm, and temperature 36.5°C. F.N. reports that her pain with uterine contractions is 6/10, located in her back and lower pelvis.

When you receive hand-off regarding F.N.'s care, her cervix has progressed to 5 cm dilation, 100% effacement, with the fetal vertex at 0 station. F.N. has an epidural in place for labor analgesia.

The FHR tracing, shown in Figure 14.1, was obtained by cardiotachometer and tocodynamometer and is what you see as you assume care of F.N.

1. Reviewing columns 01 through 30, F.N.'s uterine contractions are described best as:

    A. every two to four minutes, lasting 70 to 140 seconds, with intensity to be determined by palpation.
    B. every one to two minutes, lasting 70 to 80 seconds, with a peak intensity of 100 mmHg and a baseline uterine tone of 20 mmHg.
    C. every three minutes, lasting 50 to 60 seconds, with a peak intensity of 100 mmHg and a baseline uterine tone of 50 mmHg.
    D. every one and one-half to two and one-half minutes, lasting 80 to 100 seconds, with intensity to be determined by palpation.

2. You review F.N.'s FHR tracing and prepare to make an entry in her medical record at column 30. Your best assessment of her FHR tracing in columns 01 through 30 is:

    A. baseline FHR of 130 bpm with moderate variability (amplitude range of 6 to 25 bpm) and intermittent variable decelerations.
    B. baseline FHR of 135 bpm with minimal variability (amplitude range greater than undetectable to less than or equal to 5 bpm) and recurrent late decelerations.
    C. baseline FHR of 130 bpm with moderate variability (amplitude range of 6 to 25 bpm) and no decelerations.

3. True statement(s) regarding columns 01 through 30 of F.N.'s FHR tracing include: (Choose all that apply)

    A. This is a Category I FHR tracing.
    B. This FHR tracing is strongly predictive of normal fetal acid-base status.
    C. This FHR tracing can be followed in a routine manner.
    D. The tocodynamometer should be readjusted.

4. Select the correct statement(s) regarding FHR variability.

    A. Moderate baseline FHR variability reliably predicts the absence of fetal metabolic acidemia at the time it is observed.
    B. Minimal or absent FHR variability alone predicts the presence of fetal hypoxemia or metabolic acidemia.
    C. Both A and B are correct.
    D. Neither A nor B are correct.

5. F.N.'s contraction pattern in columns 01 through 30 is:

    A. normal.
    B. tachysystole.

Figure 14.1

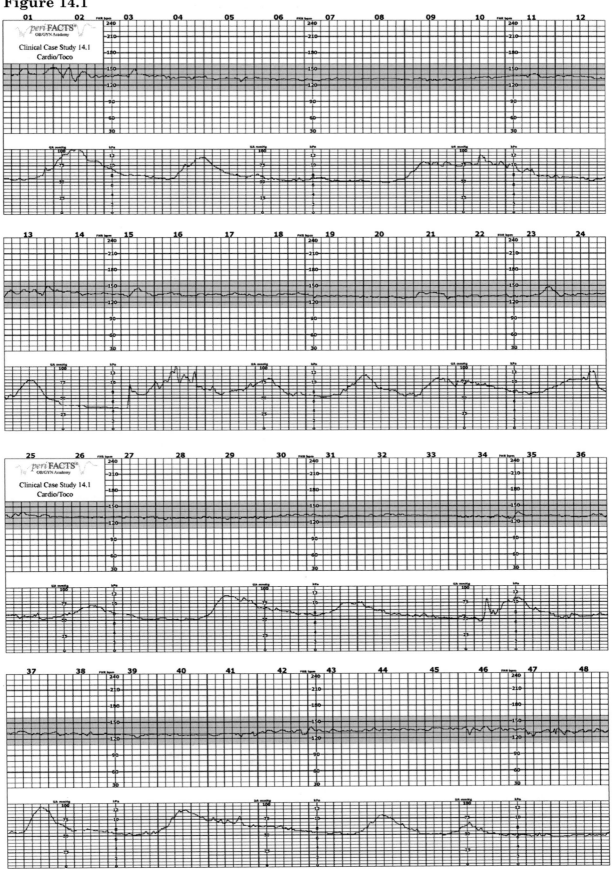

Clinical Case Study 14.1
Answers

1. The correct answer is A.

2. The correct answer is C.

3. The correct answer is A, B, C, and D.

4. The correct answer is A.

5. The correct answer is A.

OUTCOME

F.N. progresses to full dilation and has a two and one-half hour second stage of labor. F.N. spontaneously delivers a 3,350-gm female infant with Apgar scores of 8 and 9 at one and five minutes, respectively. F.N. requests and has immediate skin-to-skin contact with her newborn. Placental delivery is unremarkable, and blood loss is within normal limits. F.N. and her baby girl are discharged home on postpartum day two.

Clinical Case Study 14.2

A.B. arrives at your unit for induction in the early morning. She appears tense and is very quiet. She is accompanied by her sister and mother who are arguing with each other upon arrival. You ask her mother and sister to leave the room while you complete the admission history with A.B. and suggest that they get something to eat, giving them directions to the cafeteria.

Your admission history reveals that A.B. is a G7 P2042 woman at 41 3/7 weeks' gestation. A.B. was a late registrant to care at 24 weeks' gestation. Her dating was done with an ultrasound at 24 1/7 weeks and was consistent with her last menstrual period. She has had two previous vaginal deliveries without incident, one "natural" and one induced. Her two previous babies weighed 3,665 gm and 4,091 gm. She expresses anxiety about the induction process, stating that her pain was "much worse with the induced labor." You reassure A.B. that pain is something that can be managed with comfort measures and/or medication as she progresses in labor.

You review A.B.'s prenatal record for pregnancy risks and laboratory values. A.B.'s blood type is O positive. She is rubella immune, group B *Streptococcus* positive, and human immunodeficiency virus (HIV) and hepatitis B negative. She has no known drug allergies and uses tobacco.

The plan is to start oxytocin since her cervix is already 3 to 4 cm dilated and 40% to 50% effaced. A.B. agrees to the plan and an intravenous line is inserted, and laboratory tests are ordered. She is placed on the external fetal monitor as her family returns to the room.

Oxytocin is started, and A.B.'s amniotic membranes are ruptured, revealing meconium-stained fluid. She begins contracting almost immediately after the oxytocin is started. She becomes quite uncomfortable and refuses to let you increase the oxytocin unless she is given an epidural. An epidural is placed without incident, and A.B. rests comfortably.

1.   In the same segment of the FHR tracing, you document A.B.'s uterine contractions as:

   A.   every seven to eight minutes, because that is where the FHR decelerations occur, lasting 50 to 60 seconds, and moderate in intensity to palpation.
   B.   unable to be determined in this portion of the FHR tracing.
   C.   every four to eight minutes, lasting 50 to 60 seconds, and moderate in intensity to palpation.
   D.   one contraction in this segment of the FHR tracing, lasting 30 seconds, and moderate in intensity to palpation.

2.   You prepare to make an entry into the electronic medical record at 1500 hours. You are reviewing the FHR tracing in columns 01 to 22. You document the FHR as:

   A.   baseline FHR of 180 bpm with moderate variability (amplitude range of 6 to 25 bpm), variable and late decelerations, and no accelerations.
   B.   baseline FHR of 175 bpm with moderate variability (amplitude range of 6 to 25 bpm), variable decelerations, decelerations of unknown type, and no accelerations.
   C.   baseline FHR of 170 bpm with minimal variability (amplitude range greater than undetectable to less than or equal to 5 bpm), variable decelerations, and one acceleration.

D.   baseline FHR of 175 bpm with moderate variability (amplitude range of 6 to 25 bpm), variable and late decelerations, and no accelerations.

3.   Select the correct statement(s) regarding late FHR decelerations. (Choose all that apply.)

A.   The depth of the late FHR deceleration is indicative of the degree of fetal hypoxia.
B.   Decreased fetal PO_2 and catecholamines from the adrenal gland stimulate the vagus nerve which, in turn, causes slowing of the FHR in a late deceleration.
C.   Late FHR decelerations are associated with an increased risk of hypoxia and acidosis at birth.
D.   Late FHR decelerations are delayed in timing with the nadir of the deceleration occurring with the peak of the contraction.
E.   Late FHR decelerations can be transient in nature and resolve with resuscitative measures.
F.   Recurrent late FHR decelerations require immediate attention and intervention.

4.   Fetal tachycardia is caused by: (Choose all that are correct.)

A.   maternal fever.
B.   cigarette smoking.
C.   maternal hypothyroidism.
D.   chronic fetal hypoxemia.
E.   fetal anemia.
F.   recent illicit drug use.

5.   True or False. This FHR tracing is classified as Category III due to fetal tachycardia and late decelerations.

A.   True
B.   False

Figure 14.2

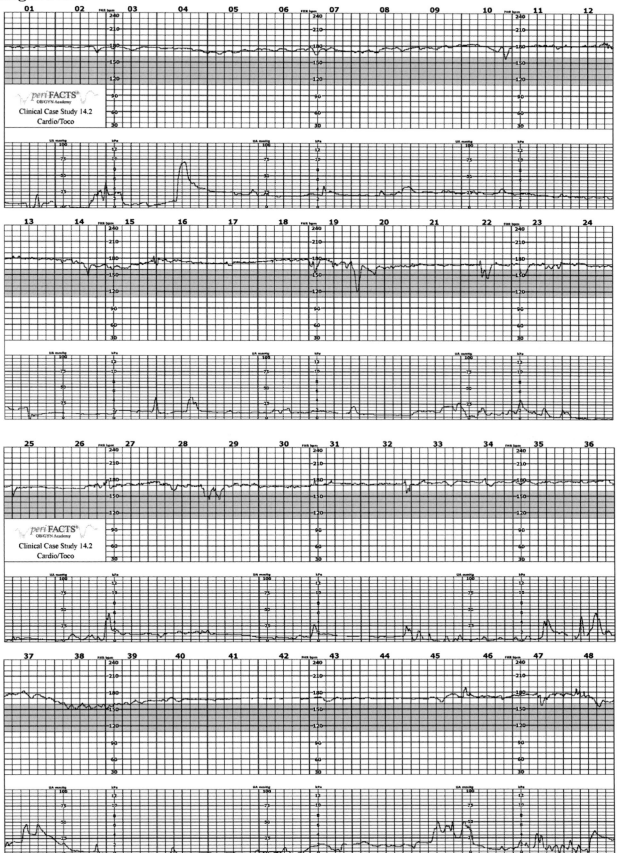

Clinical Case Study 14.2
Answers

1.   The correct answer is B.

2.   The correct answer is B. Early or late FHR decelerations require documentation of uterine contractions.

3.   The correct answer is B, C, E, and F.

4.   The correct answer is A, B, D, E, and F.

5.   The correct answer is B.

OUTCOME

Shortly after the end of this segment of the fetal heart rate tracing, A.B.'s fetus has a prolonged deceleration. Intrauterine resuscitative measures are unsuccessful, and she is taken to the operating room for an emergent cesarean section. She is able to be awake for the birth of her daughter due to a recent epidural bolus. The baby is handed to awaiting neonatal intensive care unit personnel. The baby cries spontaneously and is dried and stimulated. The baby's Apgar scores are 9 and 9 at one and five minutes, respectively. Umbilical cord blood gas samples are obtained and sent for analysis, which reveal a mild, transient respiratory acidosis. A.B.'s postoperative course is uneventful, and she and her baby are discharged home on postoperative day three in stable condition.

Clinical Case Study 14.3

F.R. is a 27-year-old, G2 P1001 woman at 40 5/7 weeks' gestation who arrives at the labor floor after contracting at home for several hours. She arrives in triage for evaluation with her husband at her side.

F.R.'s cervical examination shows her cervix to be 4 cm dilated and 80% effaced with the fetal vertex at -1 station. F.R.'s amniotic membranes are intact. She is breathing through her uterine contractions and rates her pain as a 6/10. The decision is made to admit F.R. to the labor floor for expectant management, anticipating a spontaneous vaginal delivery.

F.R.'s prenatal history is as follows.

- No significant medical history
- Appendectomy four years ago
- No known drug allergies
- Blood type O positive, rubella immune, and group B *Streptococcus* negative
- Denies alcohol, drug, and tobacco use
- Spontaneous vaginal delivery two years ago without issue

Upon admission, F.R.'s vital signs are all within normal limits.

After admission to the labor floor, she requests an epidural for pain relief. An epidural is placed for pain control. F.R. now is quite comfortable and rates her pain at 0/10. Her amniotic membranes are artificially ruptured for clear fluid. Shortly after artificial rupture of membranes, it becomes difficult to obtain a fetal heart rate tracing for F.R.'s fetus, and a fetal scalp electrode is placed to facilitate better monitoring.

F.R.'s latest cervical examination reveals her cervix to be 6 cm dilated and 100% effaced with the fetal vertex at 0 station.

F.R.'s FHR tracing is obtained by fetal scalp electrode and tocodynamometer.

1.   Your interpretation of the FHR tracing in columns 20 through 42 is:

   A.   baseline of 130 bpm with moderate variability (amplitude range of 6 to 25 bpm), periodic variable decelerations, and uterine contractions of moderate intensity occurring every four to five minutes, lasting 60 to 80 seconds.
   B.   baseline of 125 bpm with moderate variability (amplitude range of 6 to 25 bpm), recurrent variable decelerations, and uterine contractions of moderate intensity every three to five minutes, lasting 70 to 120 seconds.
   C.   baseline of 150 bpm with marked variability (amplitude range of greater than 25 bpm), recurrent decelerations, and uterine contractions of moderate intensity every three-and-a-half to five minutes, lasting 80 to 120 seconds.
   D.   baseline of 130 bpm with moderate variability (amplitude range of 6 to 25 bpm), recurrent variable decelerations, and uterine contractions of moderate intensity every four to five minutes, lasting 80 to 120 seconds.

2.   The following interventions are appropriate for this same segment of the FHR tracing. (Choose all that apply.)

   A.   Reposition the patient.
   B.   Administer an intravenous fluid bolus.
   C.   Administer oxygen via nonrebreather facemask.
   D.   Start amnioinfusion.
   E.   Perform a vaginal examination to rule out umbilical cord prolapse.

3.   Choose the true statement(s) regarding variable FHR decelerations. (Choose all that apply.)

   A.   Variable FHR decelerations generally are well tolerated by a healthy fetus.
   B.   Variable FHR decelerations are indicative of abnormal acid/base fetal status.
   C.   Variable FHR decelerations are viewed as a normal physiologic response to umbilical cord compression.
   D.   Variable FHR decelerations are the most common decelerations observed in labor.

4.   True or False. In FHR tracings with recurrent variable decelerations, the most important measure of fetal status is baseline variability.

   A.   True
   B.   False

5.   Recurrent variable FHR decelerations often lead to a transient respiratory acidosis of the fetus during labor. Which of the following fetal blood gas values reflect respiratory acidosis?

   A.   Decreased pH, increased PCO_2, decreased HCO_3-, and increased base excess.
   B.   Decreased pH, increased PCO_2, normal HCO_3-, and normal base excess.
   C.   Decreased pH, normal PCO_2, decreased HCO_3-, and increased base excess.

Figure 14.3

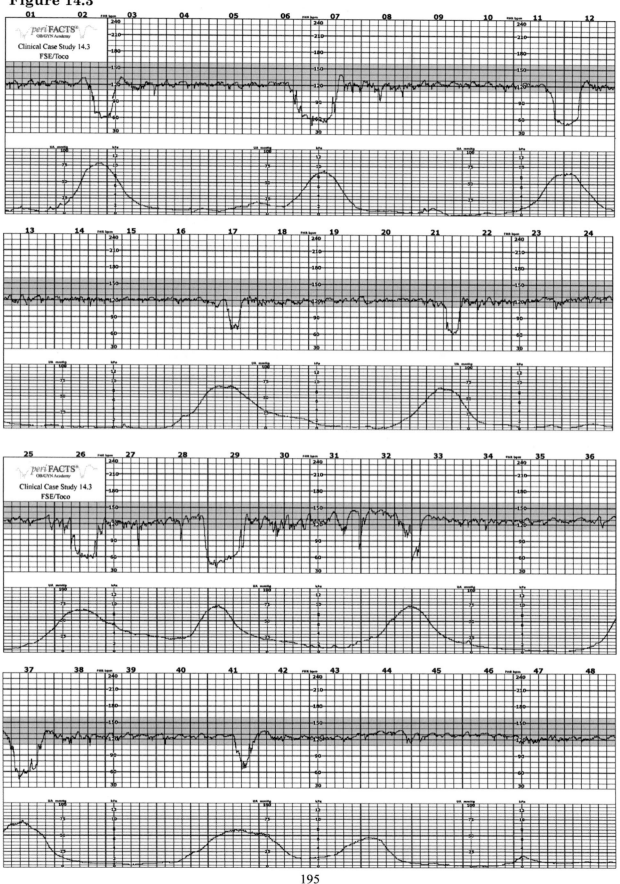

Clinical Case Study 14.3
Answers

1.   The correct answer is B.

2.   The correct answer is A, B, C, D and E.

3.   The correct answer is A, C, and D.

4.   The correct answer is A.

5.   The correct answer is B.

OUTCOME

Based on this FHR pattern, the following interventions are implemented: repositioning of the patient, providing oxygen via nonrebreather facemask, administration of an intravenous fluid bolus, amnioinfusion, and a vaginal examination to rule out umbilical cord prolapse. The fetal heart rate improves.

Approximately 20 minutes after this portion of the FHR tracing, F.R. has a normal spontaneous vaginal delivery of a viable male infant. She sustains a second-degree perineal laceration that is repaired without issue. F.R.'s baby boy requires vigorous stimulation for approximately 15 seconds before taking his first breath but is pink and vigorous at one minute with resulting Apgar scores of 7 and 9 at one and five minutes, respectively. Umbilical cord blood gas results show a mild respiratory acidosis. F.R. and her baby are discharged home on postpartum day two in stable condition.

Clinical Case Study 14.4

M.C. is a 26-year-old, G2 P1001 woman at 40 6/7 weeks' gestation by early ultrasound who presents to your obstetric triage with complaints of a large gush of fluid occurring approximately two hours ago. She has a known history of postpartum depression, successfully treated with sertraline. She reports having felt one or two uterine contractions, denies vaginal bleeding, and reports positive fetal movement.

M.C. has had one term spontaneous vaginal delivery of a 3,500-gm baby, for which she received an epidural for labor analgesia.

M.C.'s current pregnancy has been further complicated by obesity with a body mass index (BMI) of 34 kg/m² and polyhydramnios earlier in pregnancy which subsequently has resolved. She abruptly discontinued antidepressant therapy at the start of her current pregnancy. Her group B *Streptococcus* culture is negative, and she is Rh positive and Rubella immune. A one-hour glucose tolerance test shows results within normal limits. She has no other significant medical or surgical history of note. M.C. reports no drug, environmental, food, or latex allergies. She denies the use of cigarettes, alcohol, and recreational drugs.

M.C.'s medications during pregnancy include prenatal vitamins. She uses an abdominal maternity support belt.

M.C.'s most recent vital signs are: blood pressure 124/77 mmHg, pulse 86 bpm, respirations 16 rpm, and temperature 36.7°C. A sterile speculum examination is significant for positive pooling, positive nitrazine, and positive ferning, confirming that M.C.'s amniotic membranes are ruptured. Her cervical examination reveals her cervix to be 3 cm dilated, 50% effaced, with the presenting fetal part at -3 station. The estimated fetal weight of M.C.'s baby is 3,600 gm by Leopold maneuvers. Cephalic fetal presentation is confirmed by ultrasound examination.

M.C. has a saline lock placed and a type and screen with complete blood count drawn and sent for testing.

Based on her clinical presentation of spontaneous rupture of membranes, the decision is made to admit M.C. to your labor and delivery unit.

M.C. would like to receive an epidural for labor analgesia when in active labor. The provider who admitted M.C. has counseled her on the potential need for an oxytocin infusion for labor augmentation in the event of arrested cervical dilation.

The FHR tracing in Figure 14.4, obtained by cardiotachometer and tocodynamometer, is what you see as you assume care of M.C.

1. In columns 03 to 14, you would document the presence of M.C.'s uterine contractions as:

    A. occurring every two to four minutes, lasting 50 to 80 seconds, with strength to be determined by palpation.

    B. occurring every two to four-and-one-half minutes, lasting 50 to 100 seconds, with strength to be determined by palpation.

C. occurring every two to three minutes, lasting 40 to 90 seconds, with intensity of 40 to 70 mmHg above a baseline uterine resting tone of 30 mmHg.

2. In columns 01 to 17, your best interpretation of M.C.'s fetal heart rate would include:

A. FHR baseline of 145 bpm and moderate variability (amplitude range of 6 to 25 bpm) with accelerations and variable decelerations present.

B. FHR baseline of 150 bpm, moderate variability (amplitude range of 6 to 25 bpm), no accelerations, and variable and late decelerations present.

C. FHR baseline of 145 bpm, minimal variability (amplitude range greater than undetectable to less than or equal to 5 bpm) with no accelerations and variable decelerations present.

3. The pattern of frequency of the FHR decelerations occurring in M.C.'s FHR tracing is described best as:

A. recurrent.
B. intermittent.
C. episodic.

4. M.C.'s labor progresses and she undergoes an amnioinfusion. What is the indication for her amnioinfusion?

A. Variable FHR decelerations
B. Presence of meconium
C. Oligohydramnios

5. True or False. Fetal heart rate variability is the product of integrated activity between the more immature sympathetic and more mature parasympathetic branches of the autonomic nervous system.

A. True
B. False

Figure 14.4

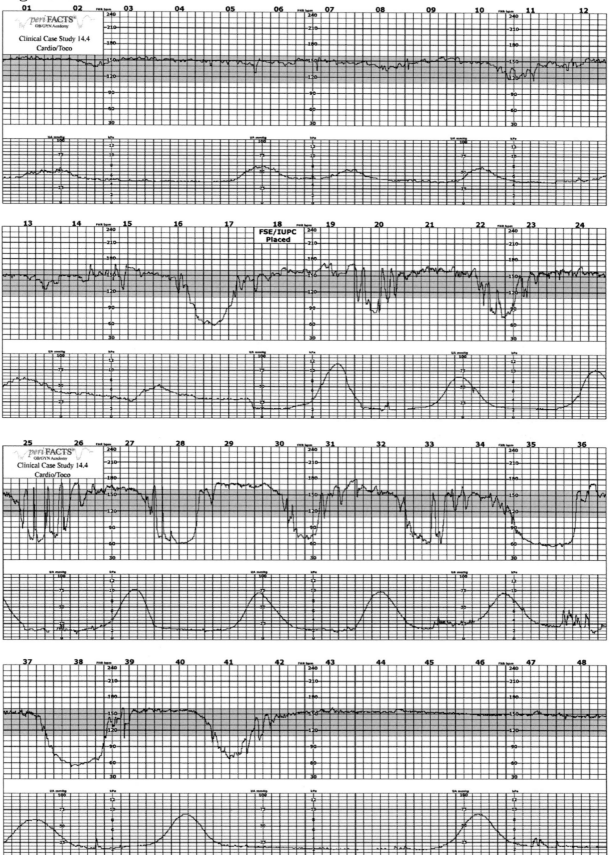

Clinical Case Study 14.4
Answers

1.   The correct answer is A.

2.   The correct answer is B.

3.   The correct answer is A.

4.   The correct answer is A.

5.   The correct answer is A.

OUTCOME

M.C. receives an epidural for labor analgesia, her cervix progresses to 5 cm dilation, and she is noted to have deep recurrent variable FHR decelerations. Intrauterine resuscitation measures are implemented including repositioning, fluid bolus, and intrauterine pressure catheter placement followed by amnioinfusion. A fetal scalp electrode is placed. The recurrent FHR variable decelerations continue despite intrauterine resuscitation interventions. Therefore, the decision is made to proceed with an urgent surgical delivery for fetal intolerance of labor. M.C. undergoes a primary low transverse cesarean section with epidural anesthesia for delivery of a viable male infant weighing 3,800 gm with Apgar scores of 8 and 9 at one and five minutes, respectively. At delivery, the umbilical cord was noted to be wrapped around the fetal neck twice. Given M.C.'s medical history of postpartum depression, including her abrupt cessation of an antidepressant upon learning of her current pregnancy, she is restarted prophylactically on sertraline in the early postpartum period prior to her discharge from your facility.

Clinical Case Study 14.5

R.K. arrives at your labor and delivery unit stating, "I'm here for my induction." She is being induced due to a post-term pregnancy. Today, R.K. is at 41 3/7 weeks' gestation by her last menstrual period, which is consistent with a five-week ultrasound. R.K. is excited and nervous. She is accompanied by three members of her immediate family and her partner. As the nurse assigned to her today, you show them all to her labor room. You orient R.K. to the use of the call bell, TV, and bed controls. You instruct her to change into a hospital gown and state you will return to get things started.

You review R.K.'s prenatal record. You learn that she is a G1 P0000 woman with an uncomplicated pregnancy. Her medical history is negative except for anemia in pregnancy. R.K. has had two surgical procedures: to repair an Achilles tendon injury and an appendectomy. She has no known drug allergies and she denies a history of smoking or use of alcohol or illicit drugs. R.K.'s blood type is O positive. She is rubella immune. She is negative for all of the following: group B *Streptococcus*, rapid plasma reagin (RPR), human immunodeficiency virus (HIV), and hepatitis B surface antigen. Her one-hour glucola is 99 mg/dL.

You return to the room and place R.K. on the electronic fetal monitor after an explanation of why this is needed during the induction process. R.K. verbalizes understanding. After 20 minutes of a reactive fetal heart rate tracing, the resident comes into the room to admit the patient. A bedside ultrasound is performed and confirms a vertex presentation. The initial cervical examination shows R.K.'s cervix to be 1.5 cm dilated, 40% effaced, with the fetal vertex at -3 station. The resident talks with R.K. about the induction process, explaining that first she will receive a "ripening" agent known as misoprostol. The resident emphasizes that this can be a long process to establish a good labor pattern. R.K. verbalizes understanding. An intravenous (IV) saline lock is inserted without difficulty, and admission laboratory specimens are drawn and sent.

Initially, R.K. is slightly bored as she remains fairly comfortable feeling only a twinge every now and then. Over the course of eight hours she becomes increasingly more uncomfortable and requests an epidural for pain relief. Her cervix at this point is 3 cm dilated and 90% effaced. The presenting fetal vertex is at -1 station. An epidural is placed with good relief. Shortly after the epidural is placed, R.K.'s amniotic membranes rupture spontaneously for a small amount of clear fluid. Labor continues to progress slowly, and it is decided to augment her labor with an oxytocin infusion. To better trace R.K.'s contractions and fetal heart rate, an intrauterine pressure catheter (IUPC) and fetal scalp electrode (FSE) are placed.

At 0100 hours, R.K.'s cervix is 8 cm dilated, 100% effaced, and the fetal vertex is at +1 station. She remains comfortable with the epidural infusion but does state that she is beginning to feel some "pressure down there." At 0300 hours, R.K. complains of increased pressure. At this time, her cervix is fully dilated, 100% effaced, and the fetal vertex is at +1 station. Because she can feel rectal pressure, she is encouraged to start pushing with the contractions. She is coached by the nurse in pushing techniques.

1.   Your assessment of the uterine contraction pattern for the entire FHR tracing is:

   A.   contractions every one to three minutes, lasting 60 to 90 seconds, with intensity to be determined by palpation.

B.   contractions every one to two minutes, lasting 50 to 80 seconds, with peak contractions of 80 mmHg above a baseline resting tone of 20 mmHg.

C.   contractions every two to three minutes, lasting 60 to 90 seconds, with peak contractions of 90 mmHg above a baseline resting tone of 15 mmHg.

D.   contractions every one and one-half to four minutes, lasting 60 to 100 seconds, with intensity to be determined by palpation.

2.   You prepare to make an entry into the electronic medical record after reviewing the entire FHR tracing. Your best interpretation of the tracing is:

A.   baseline of 145 bpm, moderate variability (amplitude range of 6 to 25 bpm), with accelerations and early FHR decelerations present.

B.   baseline of 140 bpm with moderate variability (amplitude range of 6 to 25 bpm), no accelerations, and variable FHR decelerations present.

C   baseline of 140 bpm with moderate variability (amplitude range of 6 to 25 bpm), accelerations, and early FHR decelerations present.

D.   baseline of 145 bpm with minimal variability (amplitude range greater than undetectable to less than or equal to 5 bpm), and variable and early FHR decelerations present.

3.   Overall, this FHR tracing can be categorized as:

A.   Category I.
B.   Category II.
C.   Category III.

4.   True or False. When using an FSE, the FSE mode results in counting the interval between the R waves of the fetus' QRS complex.

A.   True
B.   False

5.   When using an IUPC, an "adequate" uterine contraction generally is ____ mmHg to ____ mmHg above baseline at the peak of the contraction.

A.   20 / 60
B.   20 / 80
C.   40 / 60
D.   40 / 80

Figure 14.5

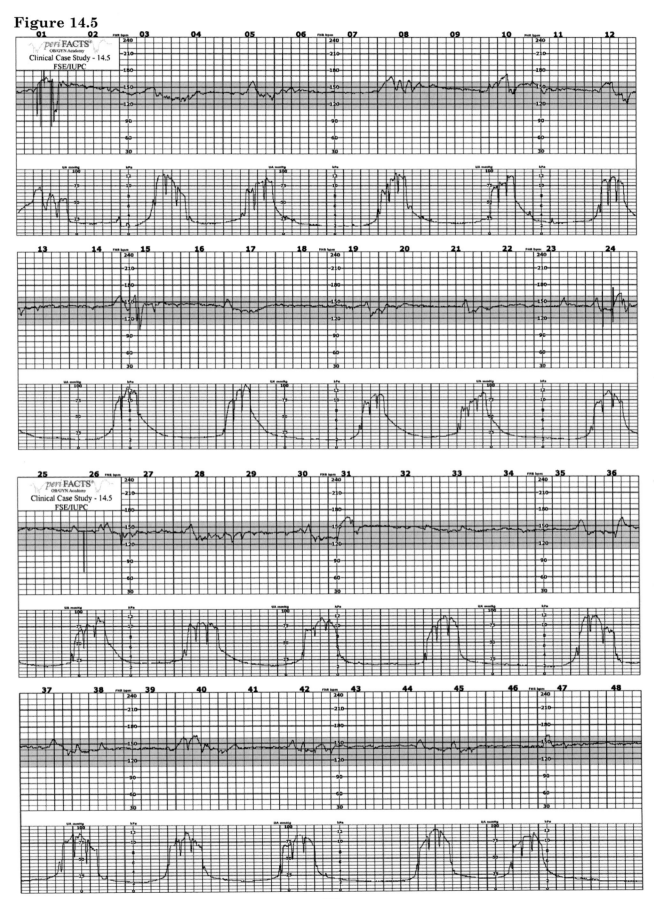

Clinical Case Study 14.5
Answers

1.   The correct answer is C.

2.   The correct answer is D.

3.   The correct answer is B.

4.   The correct answer is A.

5.   The correct answer is C.

OUTCOME

R.K. proceeds to full dilation and pushes for a total of four and a half hours. She spontaneously delivers a viable female infant weighing 3,800 gm with Apgar scores of 8 and 9 at one and five minutes, respectively. The infant is placed skin to skin with R.K., and she initiates breastfeeding immediately following delivery. Delivery resulted in a second-degree laceration, which is easily repaired. R.K. and her baby are discharged home on postpartum day two in stable condition.

Chapter 15

Advanced Fetal Heart Rate Interpretation

Clinical Case Study 15.1

C.T. presents to the triage area at 0500 hours with complaints of uterine contractions every three to four minutes for the past two hours. C.T. is a 38-year-old, G7 P5015 woman at 39 and 2/7 weeks' gestation by early ultrasound dating. She states that she has not been able to sleep through her uterine contractions, and she appears uncomfortable. She is using special breathing techniques. She denies loss of fluid, vaginal bleeding, and decreased fetal movement. C.T. is placed on the electronic fetal monitor for fetal surveillance. You recognize that C.T. does not speak English well, and you suggest using the "translator phone" for the rest of her history. C.T. initially is reluctant to use the translator phone but then agrees.

C.T. emigrated from Tanzania to escape the violence there. She delivered her first three children in Tanzania; the father of these children was killed in the violence. Initially, she sought care for termination of this pregnancy, because she is human immunodeficiency virus (HIV) positive, which was diagnosed with her last pregnancy. C.T. had been receiving antiretroviral treatment with complera, which was changed to atazanavir, emtricitabine, and ritonavir when she was found to be pregnant. C.T.'s HIV-positive status is a "social secret." None of her family members is aware of her diagnosis, although her partner is aware, and he also is HIV positive. Her partner is the father of her previous child who is HIV negative.

After her initial visit with a provider and a discussion of her non-detectable viral load and normal CD4 levels, C.T. decided to proceed with the pregnancy and plans on a bilateral tubal ligation postpartum.

Prenatal laboratory results are as follows.

- Blood type AB positive
- Rubella immune
- Syphilis screen negative
- Group B *Streptococcus* (GBS) negative
- HBsAg negative
- Hepatitis C negative
- Viral load undetectable
- CD4 of 491 two weeks ago
- One-hour glucola 125 mg/dL
- Chlamydia and gonorrhea negative

A vaginal speculum examination is performed due to a history of herpes simplex virus (HSV) infection, and no lesions are found to be present. A vaginal examination is then performed, and C.T. is found to be 4 cm dilated. Because of her HIV status and the fact that she is a grand multiparous woman, C.T. is admitted for observation of labor. An intravenous (IV) line is placed and admission laboratory samples are drawn and sent, including complete blood count, type and screen, and syphilis screen. Azidothymidine (AZT) is ordered with a loading dose of 2 mg/kg/hr followed by infusion at 1 mg/kg/hr until delivery. C.T. asks that the label for the AZT be covered, because she is expecting her sister for labor support.

You accompany C.T. to a labor room on the high-risk labor unit, settle her into the room, and give a bedside report to the next nurse who will care for her.

The fetal heart rate (FHR) tracing seen in Figure 15.1 was obtained by cardiotachometer and tocodynamometer.

1.   As you prepare to make an entry in C.T.'s record, you review her FHR tracing in columns 01 through 25. You document the uterine contractions as:

    A.   every three minutes, lasting 40 to 60 seconds, with strength to be determined by palpation.

    B.   every three to five minutes, lasting 50 to 70 seconds, with strength measured as 35 mmHg to 45 mmHg above a baseline uterine resting tone of 20 mmHg.

    C.   every two-and-one-half to four-and-one-half minutes, lasting 40 to 70 seconds, with strength to be determined by palpation.

    D.   every two-and-one-half to four minutes, lasting 50 to 60 seconds, with strength measured as 35 mmHg to 45 mmHg above a baseline uterine resting tone of 20 mmHg.

2.   In the same section of C.T.'s FHR tracing, you would document the following in the electronic medical record.

    A.   The FHR baseline is 130 bpm with moderate variability (amplitude range of 6 to 25 bpm), variable decelerations, and no accelerations present.

    B.   The FHR baseline is 125 bpm with moderate variability (amplitude range of 6 to 25 bpm), no accelerations, and variable decelerations present.

    C.   The FHR baseline is 135 bpm with minimal variability (amplitude range greater than undetectable to 5 bpm), variable decelerations, and one acceleration present.

    D.   The FHR baseline is 130 bpm with moderate variability (amplitude range of 6 to 25 bpm), no accelerations, and late decelerations present.

3.   True or False. As you continue to care for C.T., you examine her FHR tracing in columns 18 through 48. In this section of her tracing, you note that the uterine contractions show tachysystole.

    A.   True
    B.   False

4.   Causes of FHR bradycardia include: (Choose all that are correct.)

    A.   maternal hypothermia.
    B.   maternal medication response.
    C.   maternal connective tissue diseases.
    D.   decompensating fetus.
    E.   prolonged fetal sympathetic stimulation.
    F.   maternal prolonged hyperglycemia.
    G.   fetal cardiac conduction defects.

5. After you review C.T.'s FHR tracing in columns 35 through 47, when C.T.'s cervix is 5 cm dilated, you determine the nursing resuscitation measures needed would include:

    A. IV fluid bolus.
    B. maternal position change.
    C. vaginal examination to check for prolapsed umbilical cord.
    D. all of the above.
    E. B and C only.

6. True or False. Placement of a fetal scalp electrode is indicated for C.T. to more accurately record her FHR.

    A. True
    B. False

Figure 15.1

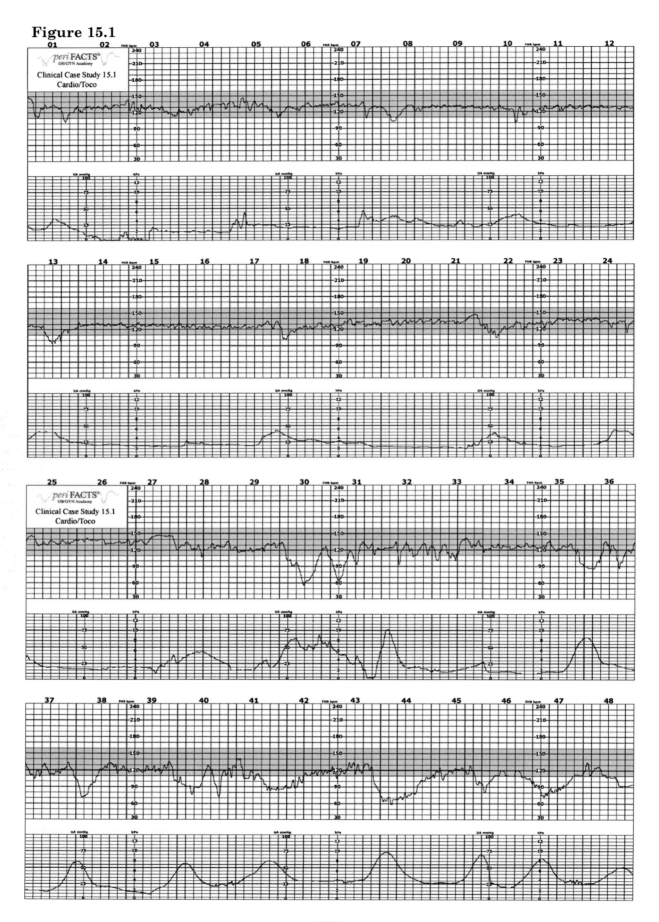

Clinical Case Study 15.1
Answers

1.   The correct answer is C.

2.   The correct answer is A.

3.   The correct answer is B.

4.   The correct answer is A, B, C, D, and G.

5.   The correct answer is D.

6.   The correct answer is B. The general recommendation is to avoid internal monitoring if at all possible due to increased risk of HIV transmission to the fetus.

OUTCOME

C.T. continues to labor with recurrent variable FHR decelerations, despite frequent position changes, oxygen via nonrebreather facemask, and intravenous fluid boluses. A cervical examination shows her cervix to be 6 cm dilated. One minute after the end of this FHR tracing, the decision is made to proceed with an emergent cesarean section due to a prolonged FHR deceleration. C.T. gives verbal consent, and she is rushed to the operating room. Because of the concerning FHR status, C.T. is placed under general anesthesia. A low transverse cesarean section with bilateral tubal ligation is performed. Nonparticulate meconium is noted with artificial rupture of membranes. The newborn male delivers with Apgar scores of 6 and 9 at one and five minutes, respectively, and weighs 2,850 gm. The baby is handed to the waiting neonatal intensive care unit team and is taken to the newborn nursery for evaluation. Following the procedure, C.T. is sent to the recovery room, awake and alert. The baby is started on combination antiretroviral therapy (cART) along with zidovudine. C.T. is continued on her cART regimen. C.T. and her baby are discharged home in stable condition on postpartum day three.

Clinical Case Study 15.2

M.C. is a 34-year-old, G5 P2022 woman at 40 and 4/7 weeks' gestation who arrives at your labor and delivery unit for an induction of labor for coordination of care for her infant at the time of delivery. During M.C.'s pregnancy, a routine obstetric ultrasound revealed a suspected fetal cardiac anomaly.

Further testing, including a fetal cardiac evaluation and echocardiogram, showed dextro-transposition of the great vessels with an intact ventricular septum. M.C. met with a genetic counselor and was followed closely by pediatric cardiology and by her obstetrician for the remainder of her pregnancy.

As you admit M.C., she reports good fetal movement, no loss of amniotic fluid, no vaginal bleeding, and no uterine contractions.

M.C.'s past medical history is significant for psoriasis. She reports no drug, food, or latex allergies. She further denies the use of cigarettes, smokeless tobacco, alcohol, and recreational drugs.

M.C. takes a prenatal vitamin daily.

M.C.'s prenatal laboratory results are:

- blood type A positive,
- group B *Streptococcus* negative,
- human immunodeficiency virus (HIV) nonreactive, and
- hepatitis B surface antigen (HBsAg) negative.

The estimated fetal weight of M.C.'s baby is 3,791 gm, and a vertex presentation is confirmed by ultrasound examination.

M.C.'s most recent vital signs are:

- blood pressure: 119/73 mmHg,
- pulse: 74 bpm,
- respirations: 20 rpm, and
- temperature: 36.3°C.

M.C.'s pelvic examination reveals her cervix to be fingertip dilated, thick, and the presenting fetal part is high. Her amniotic membranes are intact.

An intravenous (IV) line is started. A complete blood count (CBC), type and screen, and syphilis screen are drawn and sent to the laboratory. The induction process is discussed with M.C. and her husband. M.C.'s induction begins with a dose of vaginal misoprostol followed by placement of a cervical Foley catheter three hours later.

M.C. progresses in labor and receives an epidural for labor analgesia. Her cervix is now 8 cm dilated and 80% effaced with the presenting fetal vertex at -2 station. Her FHR tracing, obtained by cardiotachometer and tocodynamometer, is what you see in Figure 15.2.

1. Reviewing columns 25 through 48, M.C.'s uterine contractions are described best as:

   A. every one to two minutes, lasting 70 to 80 seconds, with intensity of 30 mmHg to 40 mmHg above a baseline uterine resting tone of 20 mmHg.
   B. every one-and-one-half to two-and-one-half minutes, lasting 60 to 110 seconds, with an intensity of 20 mmHg to 50 mmHg above a baseline uterine resting tone of 40 mmHg.
   C. Every one-and-one-half to two-and-one-half minutes, lasting 60 to 110 seconds, with intensity to be determined by palpation.

2. Your best assessment of M.C.'s FHR tracing in columns 25 through 48 is:

   A. baseline FHR of 155 bpm with moderate variability (amplitude range of 6 to 25 bpm), and an early deceleration.
   B. baseline FHR of 155 bpm with moderate variability (amplitude range of 6 to 25 bpm), and variable and late decelerations.
   C. baseline FHR of 155 bpm with minimal variability (amplitude range greater than undetectable to less than or equal to 5 bpm), and variable decelerations.

3. Because of differences between fetal and newborn circulations, most FHR tracings from fetuses with major cardiac anomalies present as:

   A. abnormal.
   B. normal.

4. The primary purpose of FHR monitoring is to assess:

   A. fetal cardiac structure.
   B. fetal movement.
   C. fetal oxygenation.
   D. cardiac function.

5. Select the cardiovascular events that occur after the umbilical cord is clamped. (Choose all that apply.)

   A. Ductus arteriosus begins to close.
   B. Newborn blood pressure increases.
   C. Foramen ovale begins to close.
   D. Ductus venosus begins to open.

6. You would categorize this entire FHR tracing as:

   A. Category I.
   B. Category II.
   C. Category III.

Figure 15.2

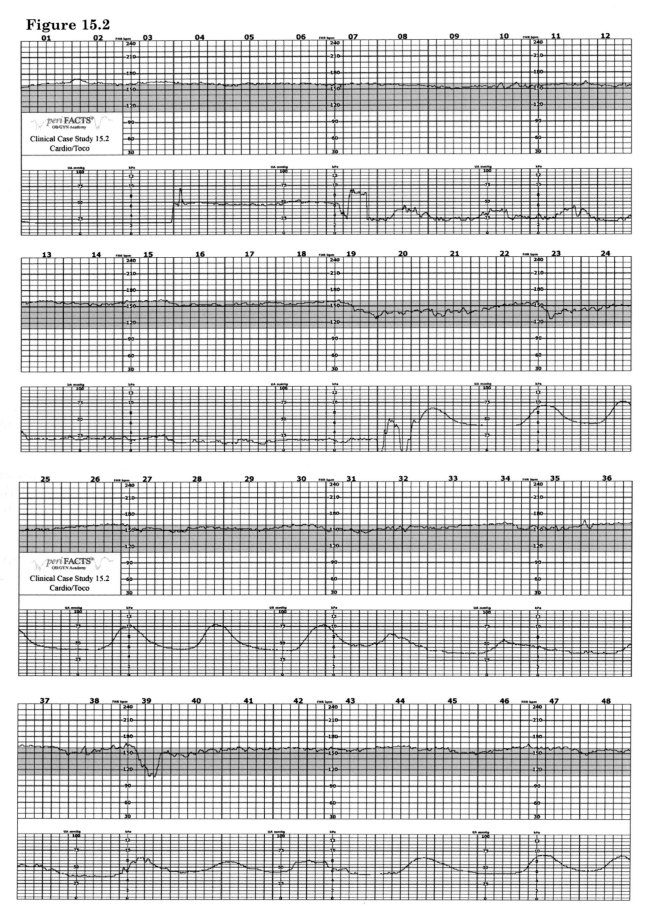

Clinical Case Study 15.2
Answers

1. The correct answer is C.

2. The correct answer is B.

3. The correct answer is B.

4. The correct answer is C.

5. The correct answer is A, B, and C.

6. The correct answer is B.

OUTCOME

M.C. progresses to full dilation and spontaneously delivers a 3,665-gm male infant. The infant is placed on M.C.'s abdomen. The umbilical cord is clamped and cut before he is handed, floppy and cyanotic, to the awaiting neonatal intensive care unit team. M.C. has a second-degree laceration, which is repaired. The estimated blood loss is 350 mL. The placenta delivers without difficulty.

Due to poor oxygen saturation levels, M.C.'s infant son is taken immediately to the operating room for an emergent balloon atrial septostomy performed by the pediatric cardiology team. He does well postoperatively and is discharged to his parents at 14 days of age to be followed by pediatric cardiology.

M.C. has an uneventful postpartum course. She is instructed on how to use a breast pump, because she plans to breastfeed her son. She is discharged home in stable condition on postpartum day three.

Clinical Case Study 15.3

M.A. is a 20-year-old, G3 P2002 woman at 24 and 1/7 weeks' estimated gestational age who presents to your labor and delivery unit with vaginal bleeding. She reports that the bleeding started five weeks earlier after she fell on her abdomen. She was advised to limit her activity due to concerns for a possible placental abruption. Her bleeding had been stable until today when it started to become heavy, and she passed eight golf ball-sized clots. M.A. also complains of mild, left-sided abdominal pain when she sits up. She called her obstetric care provider and was directed to go to your labor and delivery unit.

During M.A.'s admission process, you apply the electronic fetal monitor and note the following vital signs.

- Temperature: 36.8°C
- Pulse: 111 bpm
- Respirations: 18 rpm
- Blood pressure: 129/66 mmHg
- Pain assessment: abdominal, 2/10
- Weight: 210 lb (body mass index 33.9 kg/m^2)

M.A.'s pregnancy risks include:

- vaginal bleeding,
- preterm status, and
- low-lying placenta, 2.5 to 3 cm from the internal os.

M.A. reports that she is allergic to penicillin and doxycycline, but she denies environmental, food, or latex allergies. She further denies the use of cigarettes, alcohol, and recreational drugs.

M.A.'s medications during this pregnancy include a daily prenatal vitamin and iron.

A review of M.A.'s prenatal laboratory results are as follows.

- Blood type O positive
- Rubella IgG AB positive
- Rapid plasma reagin negative
- Hepatitis B surface antigen (HBsAg) negative
- Human immunodeficiency virus (HIV) negative

M.A. is admitted to your labor and delivery unit for expectant management of her pregnancy due to concerns for preterm labor, a placental abruption, and oligohydramnios. A sterile speculum examination reveals a closed cervix, effacement 20%, and intact amniotic membranes. A small amount of red-brown blood is observed in the vaginal vault. A fetal cephalic presentation is confirmed by a bedside ultrasound examination. Estimated weight of the fetus is 660 gm by ultrasound. An intravenous saline lock is placed and blood samples are drawn for a syphilis screen, complete blood count, Kleihauer-Betke, and a type and screen.

M.A. is consented for a cesarean section and a neonatal intensive care unit consultation is obtained. A betamethasone corticosteroid course for fetal lung maturity is ordered.

M.A continues to bleed a mild-to-moderate amount. Her hematocrit remains relatively stable in the 26% to 28% range. Her Kleihauer-Betke results are negative.

Over the course of the next several days, M.A. continues to report positive fetal movement, while she remains on continuous fetal monitoring. Intermittent uterine contractions are noted during this time period, which are difficult to trace and resolve on their own.

The FHR tracing seen in Figure 15.3, obtained by cardiotachometer and tocodynamometer, is what you see.

1.   Reviewing columns 01 through 24, M.A.'s uterine contractions are described best as:

   A.   unable to assess contractions; reapply the tocodynamometer.
   B.   every one to three-and-one-half minutes, lasting 20 to 100 seconds, with intensity of 25 mmHg above a baseline uterine resting tone of 20 mmHg.
   C.   one contraction lasting 20 seconds with intensity to be determined by palpation.
   D.   no contractions.

2.   The best assessment of M.A.'s FHR tracing in columns 01 through 24 is:

   A.   baseline FHR of 170 bpm with absent variability (amplitude range is undetectable) and recurrent late decelerations.
   B.   baseline FHR of 170 bpm with minimal variability (amplitude range greater than undetectable to less than or equal to 5 bpm), and variable decelerations.
   C.   baseline FHR of 160 bpm with moderate variability (amplitude range of 6 to 25 bpm) and variable decelerations.
   D.   baseline FHR of 160 bpm with moderate variability (amplitude range of 6 to 25 bpm) and recurrent late decelerations.

3.   When monitoring the preterm fetus in labor, it is important to remember that:

   A.   the fetus will have reduced FHR variability.
   B.   the fetus will have less reserves during times of stress.
   C.   the fetus is prone to umbilical cord compression.
   D.   all of the above.
   E.   A and B only.

4.   If a fetus becomes hypoxemic, the fetus redirects its blood volume to the following vital organs. (Choose all that apply.)

   A.   Brain
   B.   Heart
   C.   Kidneys
   D.   Adrenals

5. At the time of M.A.'s delivery, the following umbilical cord arterial blood gas values are obtained: pH 7.02, PCO_2 90 mmHg, PO_2 8 mmHg, HCO_3- 15 mEq/L, and base excess -10 mEq/L. These values are indicative of:

   A. normal umbilical vein blood gas values.
   B. respiratory acidosis.
   C. metabolic acidosis.
   D. mixed respiratory and metabolic acidosis.

6. In the second and third trimester, amniotic fluid is derived exclusively from:

   A. the fetal lung secretions.
   B. transudate of fetal plasma through skin.
   C. fetal kidneys in the form of urine.
   D. all of the above.
   E. A and C only.

Figure 15.3

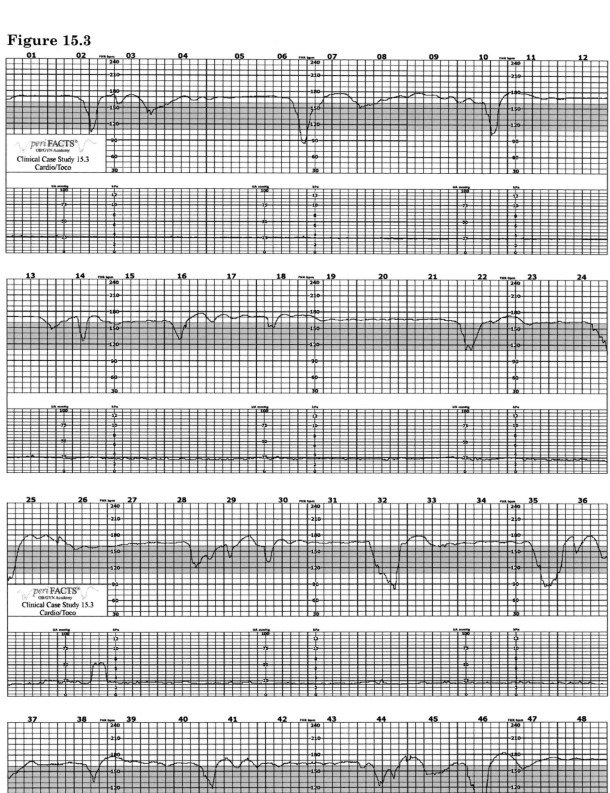

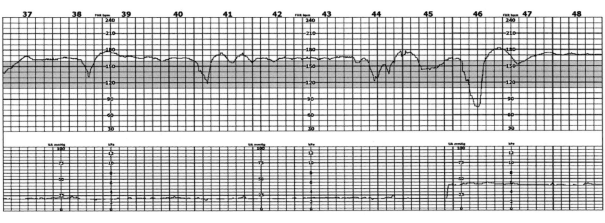

Clinical Case Study 15.3
Answers

1. The correct answer is A.

2. The correct answer is B. Without uterine contractions, one can document variable FHR decelerations but not late or early FHR decelerations.

3. The correct answer is D.

4. The correct answer is A, B, and D.

5. The correct answer is D.

6. The correct answer is E.

OUTCOME

Seven days after M.A.'s admission, while being monitored, the FHR again shows recurrent FHR decelerations. At this time, M.A. also is having uterine contractions that are not seen on the tocodynamometer but are palpable. The fetus demonstrates tachycardia with FHRs in the 180s and has recurrent, severe, variable FHR decelerations despite resuscitative efforts. During an attempt for a biophysical profile, no fetal movement is noted for six minutes. An urgent call is made to the maternal-fetal medicine backup who recommends urgent delivery. Therefore, a plan is made to move to the operating room for cesarean section.

After receiving general anesthesia, M.A. has an urgent, primary, classical, cesarean section delivery of a viable male infant in the vertex position. At the time the amniotic membranes are ruptured, particulate meconium and a small blood clot are noted in the amniotic fluid. The infant's umbilical cord is clamped and cut. The infant is handed off to the awaiting neonatal intensive care (NICU) team. The placenta, with a three-vessel umbilical cord, is removed manually, and an adherent clot is noted on the placenta. Estimated blood loss is 750 mL. M.A. tolerates the delivery well.

The baby boy, weighing 550 gm, is apneic, cyanotic, and without a heart rate. His Apgar scores are 0, 0, 0, 4, and 6 at one, five, ten, fifteen, and twenty minutes, respectively. He is resuscitated for approximately 15 minutes and intubated prior to achieving a pulse, at which time he is transferred to the NICU. The infant is small-for-gestational age, with no notable dysmorphic features and with diminished physical tone. His course is complicated by a grade 4 right intraparenchymal hemorrhage, respiratory distress syndrome, and sepsis, with a notable right hemidiaphragm. Phrenic nerve damage also is suspected, possibly occurring during his birth.

Postoperatively, M.A. does well. She meets all of her postoperative milestones and is discharged home in stable condition on postoperative day four with instructions to follow up with her obstetric care provider in seven to ten days.

M.A.'s infant son has a prolonged admission in the NICU. He is discharged with a tracheostomy, on a ventilator, to be followed by pediatric pulmonary, gastroenterology, and otolaryngology with visiting nurse services.

Clinical Case Study 15.4

Change of shift report has just finished when your unit receives a call from an outlying hospital asking to transfer a patient at 37 weeks' gestation who is in early labor in order to be nearer your institution's neonatal intensive care unit. The patient, S.B., admitted to recent heroin and cocaine use. She is aware that most likely the baby will have to stay in the hospital for management of withdrawal symptoms. You are assigned to the care of S.B. and receive a telephone report from her current nurse.

S.B. is a 25-year-old, G6 P3023 woman at 37 1/7 weeks' gestation. She has been in and out of treatment centers for her addiction to heroin, cocaine, and opioids. Earlier today, she was interviewed at a treatment center when she began to feel uterine contractions. S.B. went to the transferring hospital and was found to be in early labor. She was observed for two hours, and her cervix changed from 1 cm to 3 cm. S.B. admitted to using heroin and cocaine two nights ago and stated that she had been given oxycodone last night for pain. She also admits to taking "street suboxone" from time to time but doesn't remember the last use. S.B. has had three prior vaginal deliveries without difficulty and stated that "they were fast." She smokes cigarettes daily and has a medical history of asthma and anxiety. S.B. has no known allergies.

The nurse giving you report states that S.B.'s uterine contractions are irregular and are anywhere from ten to 15 minutes apart, lasting 40 to 60 seconds, with mild intensity by palpation. The fetal heart rate (FHR) tracing is Category I. The nurse also states that S.B. was planning an epidural for pain relief with labor but, at the time of transfer, was not uncomfortable.

An intravenous line (IV) was placed prior to transfer. The nurse states that S.B., accompanied by a nurse, left in the ambulance about ten minutes prior to her calling in the report.

You know that the ambulance trip will take approximately 40 minutes, and you go to the room to prepare for a possible quick delivery.

S.B. arrives at your facility in active labor, screaming in pain with uterine contractions, and requesting an epidural for pain relief. You assist S.B. into bed and place her on the electronic fetal monitor. The anesthesiologist is paged for a possible epidural placement, but cervical examination shows S.B.'s cervix to be 8 cm dilated. You quickly draw laboratory specimens for a type and screen and complete blood count, as well as rapid human immunodeficiency virus (HIV), hepatitis B, rubella, and syphilis testing.

While S.B. is waiting for the anesthesiologist to arrive, you obtain the FHR tracing shown in Figure 15.4 by cardiotachometer and tocodynamometer.

1.   After reviewing S.B.'s FHR tracing in columns 01 through 24, you chart the uterine contractions as:

     A.   two minutes apart, lasting 30 to 60 seconds, with moderate intensity as determined by palpation.

     B.   one to two minutes apart, lasting 50 to 70 seconds, with moderate intensity as determined by palpation.

     C.   one to two minutes apart, lasting 30 to 60 seconds, with an intensity of 40 mmHg over a baseline uterine resting tone of 5 mmHg.

D.   one to two minutes apart, lasting 30 to 60 seconds, with intensity to be determined by palpation.

2.   In this same portion of S.B.'s FHR tracing, you prepare to enter the following information into the electronic medical record.

     A.   The FHR baseline is 140 bpm with moderate variability (amplitude range of 6 to 25 bpm), accelerations, and no decelerations present.

     B.   The FHR baseline is 170 bpm with moderate variability (amplitude range of 6 to 25 bpm), and variable decelerations present.

     C.   The FHR baseline is indeterminate.

     D.   This portion of the FHR tracing has a "wandering" baseline.

3.   True or False. Baseline FHR is the average FHR over a period of ten minutes, not including periodic or episodic changes in the FHR, rounded to the nearest 5 bpm with at least two minutes of continuous, discernable baseline.

     A.   True

     B.   False

4.   A biophysical profile (BPP) consists of five measured parameters, and each parameter is given a value of 0 or 2. Based on the information below, what is the score for this BPP on a 30-week fetus with preterm premature rupture of membranes?

Biophysical Profile Results	
Nonstress Test	Reactive with two accelerations of 10 bpm and 10 seconds in duration
Fetal Breathing	One episode of 20 seconds
Fetal Movement	Three discrete movements
Fetal Tone	Two episodes of active extension of legs
Amniotic Fluid Volume	Two pockets of 1 cm of fluid

     A.   4/10

     B.   6/10

     C.   8/10

5.   When a BPP is performed, the parameter(s) most indicative of longer duration or greater severity of impaired oxygenation is/are: (Choose all that apply).

     A.   loss of fetal breathing.

     B.   loss of FHR variability.

     C.   loss of fetal tone.

     D.   loss of fetal gross body movements.

6.   Key elements to affect team communication are: (Choose all that apply.)

     A. use of common terminology.

     B. an organized structure.

     C. timely and accurate communication.

Figure 15.4

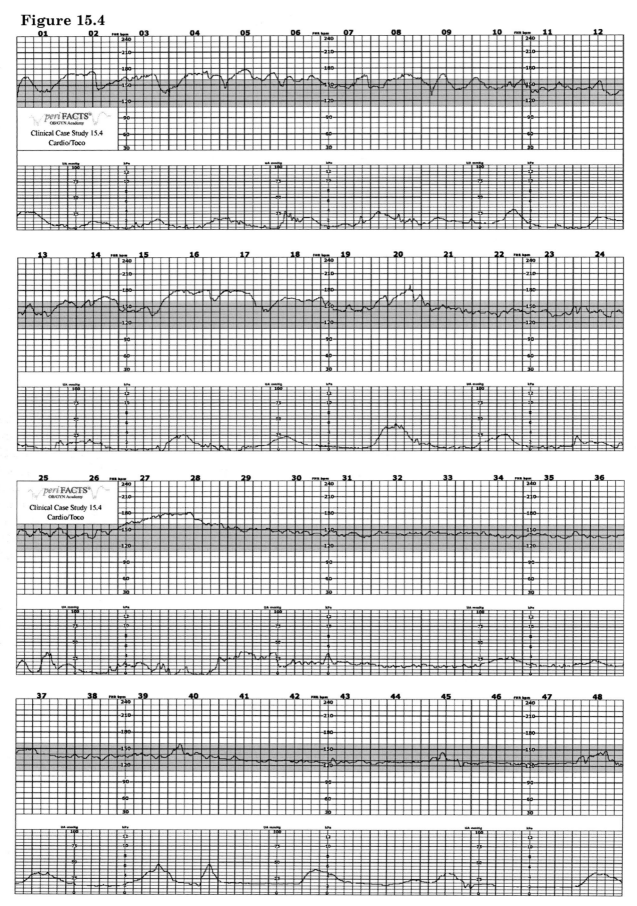

Clinical Case Study 15.4
Answers

1. The correct answer is D.

2. The correct answer is A.

3. The correct answer is B. At least two minutes of discernable FHR baseline must be present, not necessarily continuous baseline.

4. The correct answer is B. Two points each are given for reactive nonstress test, fetal movement, and fetal tone.

5. The correct answer is C and D.

6. The correct answer is A, B, and C.

OUTCOME

Anesthesia personnel arrive in S.B.'s room, and it is determined that an epidural will take too long to give her the necessary relief from her uterine contractions. A saddle block is placed and S.B. receives adequate relief. Shortly after placement of the saddle block, her amniotic membranes rupture for moderately stained meconium fluid. Anticipating a quick delivery, the neonatal intensive care unit (NICU) team had been called and are in the delivery room. S.B. precipitously delivers a female infant over an intact perineum. The baby is handed to the awaiting NICU team. Apgar scores are 7 and 9 at one and five minutes, respectively. The baby weighs 2,950 gm. The baby initially has a strong cry but shows signs of grunting and subcostal retractions by five minutes of life. She is suctioned for copious amounts of meconium and blood-tinged sputum. The decision is made to admit the newborn to the NICU for further evaluation.

S.B.'s postpartum course is uncomplicated, and she is discharged on postpartum day two after being scheduled with a rehabilitation clinic for her drug addictions. S.B.'s daughter has a prolonged hospital stay due to respiratory distress and withdrawal symptoms. She eventually is discharged on day 30 of life in stable condition to her mother's care with the involvement of Child Protective Services.

Clinical Case Study 15.5

B.T., a 25-year-old, G6 P1223 woman at 31 5/7 weeks' gestation, was at work when she noticed a small leak of clear fluid. She called her obstetric care provider who advised her to go the hospital for evaluation, because it was past office hours, and because B.T. has a history of two previous preterm deliveries due to preterm premature rupture of membranes (PPROM). Rupture of amniotic membranes is confirmed at the hospital. B.T. is placed on the electronic fetal monitor (EFM), and a reactive fetal heart rate (FHR) tracing is observed.

B.T.'s care provider recommends transfer to the tertiary care hospital down the street where there is a state-of-the-art neonatal intensive care unit (NICU). B.T. agrees to be transferred. An intravenous (IV) line is placed, latency antibiotics are started for unknown group B *Streptococcus* (GBS) status, and B.T. is given her first dose of betamethasone to facilitate fetal lung maturity while awaiting the ambulance for transfer. Upon arrival at the tertiary care center, B.T. is seen in the triage area where you have been assigned. She is placed on the EFM and several small variable FHR decelerations are seen. Admission bloodwork is drawn, and a second speculum examination is performed to confirm PPROM and obtain vaginal cultures. B.T. is somewhat annoyed by the repeat examinations and tests. She is tired after working all day and just wants to go to bed.

The maternal-fetal medicine (MFM) physician arrives to speak with B.T. and to discuss the plan with her. She is counseled on the etiologies of PPROM, risks of PPROM including infection, placental abruption, and prolapsed umbilical cord. The MFM physician also discusses the role of the NICU team. B.T. is told that the optimal timing of delivery is unknown, but at this institution, 36 weeks typically is recommended in the absence of infection or other concerns. B.T. is familiar with all of this due to her previous preterm deliveries and states understanding of the risks and plan.

A reactive FHR tracing now is observed without evidence of uterine contractions. An ultrasound confirms vertex presentation of the fetus. The decision is made to admit B.T. to the antepartum unit for continued observation where she will not need continuous EFM. B.T. is happy to finally be able to go to sleep and walks to her new room.

Before transfer to the antepartum unit, you review B.T.'s history and fill in the handoff tool in the electronic medical record (EMR).

B.T.'s pregnancy risks include:

- history of PPROM at 31 and 3/7 weeks' gestation, primary low-transverse cesarean section for concerning fetal heart rate at 33 weeks' gestation,
- history of PPROM at 33 weeks' gestation with successful vaginal birth after cesarean section at 35 weeks,
- positive fetal fibronectin test four days prior to PPROM,
- rubella non-immune,
- history of postpartum depression not requiring treatment with medication, and
- anemia.

After B.T. is tucked in "for the duration," you give face-to-face report:

B.T.'s latest vital signs are:

- blood pressure: 138/75 mmHg,
- pulse: 110 bpm,
- temperature: 36.6°C,
- respirations: 18 rpm, and
- oxygen saturation: 100%.

B.T. has been given her first dose of betamethasone. Her second dose is due at 2200 hours tomorrow. The penicillin for unknown GBS status is due at 0200 hours. An order for daily nonstress tests has been placed. B.T. is hoping to have another vaginal delivery.

Seven days later, at 32 and 5/7 weeks' gestation, B.T. calls out to the nurse on the antepartum unit with complaints of abdominal tenderness and uterine contractions. She is evaluated by the resident, and a decision is made to transfer her to the labor unit where she can be continuously monitored. B.T. now is contracting every three to five minutes. B.T.'s temperature is 38.2°C and her pulse is 112 bpm. The decision is made to move toward delivery for presumed chorioamnionitis. Antibiotics are administered, and oxytocin is started for induction of labor. A cervical examination shows her cervix to be 2 cm dilated, 50% effaced, and the fetal vertex is at -2 station.

The fetal heart rate tracing seen in Figure 15.5 is obtained with a cardiotachometer and tocodynamometer.

1.   Confusion arises about when it is appropriate to document certain aspects of an FHR tracing. Choose all of the correct statements.

    A.   Late FHR decelerations can be recorded even when uterine contractions are not being identified.
    B.   FHR variability requires establishing a stable (more than two minutes in ten minutes) FHR baseline.
    C.   Variable FHR decelerations can be documented in the absence of uterine contractions.
    D.   Early FHR decelerations require documenting uterine contractions.
    E.   Category I, II, and III designations for FHR tracings are used during the intrapartum period and may be used during the antepartum period.

2.   You review B.T.'s FHR tracing in columns 20 through 40 and prepare to enter the following interpretation in the electronic medical record.

    A.   Uterine contractions approximately two minutes apart, with strength to be determined by palpation. FHR baseline of 170 bpm with minimal variability (amplitude range greater than undetectable to less than or equal to 5 bpm), recurrent variable FHR decelerations, and no accelerations.
    B.   Unable to determine uterine contraction frequency and duration in this section of the FHR tracing. FHR baseline of 170 bpm with minimal variability (amplitude range greater than undetectable to less than or equal to 5 bpm); FHR decelerations cannot be classified, because uterine contractions are not tracing well.

C. Uterine contractions every three minutes with strength to be determined by palpation. FHR baseline of 170 bpm with minimal variability (amplitude range greater than undetectable to less than or equal to 5 bpm), variable FHR decelerations, and no accelerations.

D. Uterine contractions not tracing well; therefore, unable to determine frequency and duration. FHR baseline of 165 bpm with minimal variability (amplitude range greater than undetectable to less than or equal to 5 bpm), recurrent late decelerations, and no accelerations.

3. Match the terms below with their correct definition.

A.	Recurrent FHR decelerations	1.	Late FHR decelerations with 50% or more of contractions during a CST
B.	Episodic changes	2.	Accelerations and/or decelerations occurring with relationship to uterine contractions
C.	Periodic changes		
		3.	No late or significant variable decelerations during a CST.
D.	Positive contraction stress test (CST)		
		4.	Decelerations that occur with greater than or equal to 50% of uterine contractions in any 20-minute window.
E.	Negative CST		
		5.	Accelerations and/or decelerations occurring without relationship to uterine contractions

The FHR remains concerning despite intrauterine resuscitation attempts. The decision is made to proceed with a cesarean delivery due to the FHR changes and chorioamnionitis.

4. After delivery, umbilical cord blood gas values were obtained on B.T.'s female infant with the following results.

Cord arterial pH: 7.29	Cord venous pH: 7.32
Cord arterial PCO: 52 mmHg	Cord venous PCO: 46 mmHg
Cord arterial PO_2: 17 mmHg	Cord venous PO_2: 25 mmHg
Cord arterial BE: -2 mEq/L	Cord venous BE: -3 mEq/L

These results show:

A. respiratory acidosis.
B. metabolic acidosis.
C. mixed acidosis.
D. normal.

5.   B.T.'s baby is delivered and handed to an awaiting NICU team. She is cyanotic, floppy, with no respiratory effort. She is dried, stimulated, and warmed. At one minute of life, she remains cyanotic with weak respiratory effort, a heart rate of 60 bpm, some flexion of extremities, and grimace. The one-minute Apgar score for B.T.'s female infant is:

A.   5
B.   4
C.   6
D.   3

6.   You would categorize this FHR tracing as:

A.   Category I.
B.   Category II.
C.   Category III.

Figure 15.5

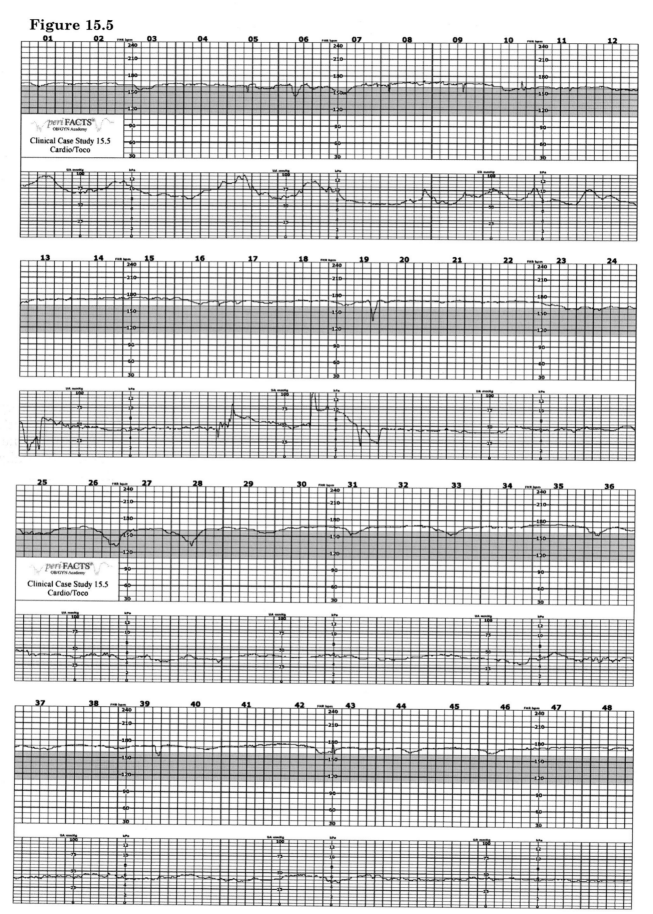

Clinical Case Study 15.5
Answers

1.   The correct answer is B, C, D, and E.

2.   The correct answer is B.

3.   The correct answer is A-4, B-5, C-2, D-1, and E-3.

4.   The correct answer is D.

5.   The correct answer is B.

6.   The correct answer is B. There is minimal FHR variability. The tocodynamometer
      needs to be adjusted.

OUTCOME

B.T.'s daughter is stabilized by the neonatal intensive care unit (NICU) team in the delivery
room. The infant's five-minute Apgar score is 8, and she is taken to the NICU. The infant's
weight is 2,185 gm. B.T. receives antibiotics for 23 hours postoperatively and remains afebrile.
She is discharged on postpartum day three meeting all postoperative milestones. Her baby
remains hospitalized for four weeks and subsequently is discharged home in stable condition.

Clinical Case Study 15.6

G.K. is a 31-year-old, G3 P1011 woman at 37 4/7 weeks' gestation by 7 1/7 weeks' ultrasound. She presents to your labor and delivery unit for a scheduled induction of labor for preeclampsia without severe features. She denies headaches, visual disturbances, and epigastric pain. She reports positive fetal movement and further denies loss of amniotic fluid and vaginal bleeding.

G.K. has a known history of chronic hypertension, obesity with a body mass index (BMI) of 56 kg/m² (175.09 kg or 386 lb), hypothyroidism, and a previous low transverse cesarean section for failure to progress in the setting of known preeclampsia. Her current pregnancy is complicated further by gestational diabetes and fetal cystic left kidney.

Upon arrival, an ultrasound is performed, which reveals an estimated fetal weight of 3,529 gm and a cephalic fetal presentation. A digital vaginal examination reveals G.K.'s cervix to be 1 cm dilated and the fetal vertex at -2 station.

You note that G.K. has an elevated 24-hour urine protein when compared to a baseline 24-hour urine collection at the start of her pregnancy. Her Group B *Streptococcus* (GBS) culture is positive, and she is Rh positive, and rubella immune. Hemolysis, elevated liver enzymes, and low platelet count syndrome (HELLP) laboratory values are within normal limits upon admission. A syphilis and human immunodeficiency virus (HIV) screen are collected. Both are negative. In addition, you collect a type and screen due to her morbid obesity as this increases her risk for a postpartum hemorrhage.

G.K. reports no medication, environmental, food, or latex allergies. Her medications during pregnancy include labetalol, 200 mg three times daily; insulin glargine, 60 units nightly; insulin lispro, 15 units three times a day with meals; levothyroxine, 50 mcg daily; aspirin, 81 mg daily; and prenatal vitamins.

G.K.'s most recent vital signs are: blood pressure 145/80 mmHg, pulse 81 bpm, respirations 18 rpm, and temperature 36.4°C. Her blood glucose level upon admission is 69 mg/dL. You plan to assess her blood glucose level every four hours during the early stage of her labor induction and increase frequency as her labor progresses to a more active stage.

You obtain intravenous access and begin administration of intravenous penicillin for a positive GBS status and magnesium sulfate for seizure prophylaxis. G.K.'s labor is induced with a cervical Foley bulb, an oxytocin infusion, and artificial rupture of amniotic membranes.

The accompanying FHR tracing, obtained by cardiotachometer and tocodynamometer, is what you see when taking G.K.'s vital signs.

1.   In columns 01 through 32, your best interpretation of G.K.'s uterine contraction pattern would include:

   A.   uterine contractions occurring every two to six and one-half minutes, lasting 50 to 70 seconds, and strength to be determined by palpation.
   B.   uterine contractions occurring every two to five minutes, lasting 50 to 70 seconds, with intensity of 30 to 40 mmHg above a baseline uterine resting tone of 5 mmHg.

C. uterine contractions occurring every two to four minutes, lasting 50 to 70 seconds, and strength to be determine by palpation.

2. In columns 01 through 32, your best interpretation of G.K.'s FHR tracing would include:

A. FHR baseline 135 bpm, moderate variability (amplitude range of 6 to 25 bpm) with accelerations and no decelerations noted.
B. FHR baseline 140 bpm, moderate variability (amplitude range of 6 to 25 bpm) with no accelerations and no decelerations noted.
C. FHR baseline 135 bpm, moderate variability (amplitude range of 6 to 25 bpm) with no accelerations and a variable deceleration noted.

3. Normal labor is a metabolic stressor on umbilical blood and gas exchange, which results in:

A. a mild decrease in fetal pH, PO_2, and bicarbonate with a mild increase in base excess.
B. a mild decrease in fetal pH and PO_2 with a mild increase in bicarbonate and base excess.
C. a mild decrease in fetal pH and bicarbonate with a mild increase in PO_2 and base excess.

4. Which of the following can be used for positioning a morbidly obese patient to perform fetal monitoring? (Choose all that apply.)

A. Pillows
B. Rolled blankets
C. Tying fetal monitoring belts together to hold fetal monitors
D. Wedges
E. Bariatric bed

5. Which of the following statements are true regarding intensity of uterine contractions?

A. Uterine contraction intensity is the magnitude of the intrauterine pressure above the baseline uterine resting tone.
B. Intrauterine pressure intensities up to 100 mmHg are not uncommon during active labor.
C. Intensity of a uterine contraction can be estimated through palpation as mild, moderate, or strong when a tocodynamometer is in use.
D. Most uterine contractions are tolerated by a healthy fetus.
E. All of the above.
F. A and D only.

6. Hemodynamic changes in pregnancy include:

A. body fluid increases to between 6.5 to 8.5 L during pregnancy.
B. plasma volume increasing by 50%, plateauing at around 33 to 34 weeks' gestation.
C. preeclampsia and bleeding both lower colloid oncotic pressure by further depleting intravascular proteins.
D. all of the above.
E. B and C only.

Figure 15.6

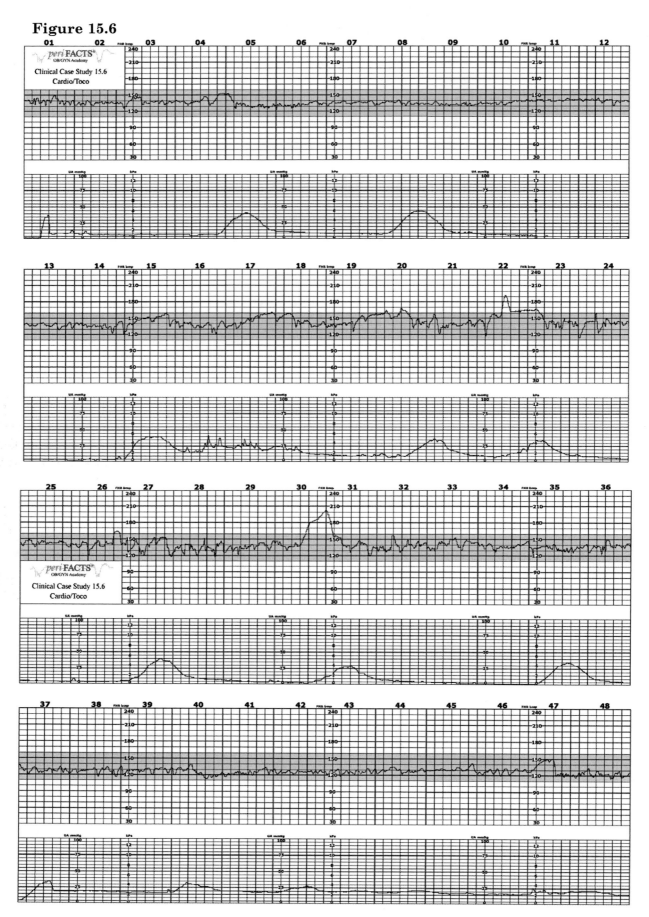

234

Clinical Case Study 15.6
Answers

1. The correct answer is A.

2. The correct answer is A.

3. The correct answer is A.

4. The correct answer is A, B, D, and E.

5. The correct answer is E.

6. The correct answer is D.

OUTCOME

At 4 cm, G.K.'s labor progression arrests, and the decision is made to proceed with an operative delivery. G.K. undergoes a repeat low transverse cesarean section under general anesthesia. It is noted that G.K. has a uterine rupture at her prior cesarean section scar on the right lateral side of the uterus measuring 3 cm in length with the amniotic sac ballooning through the myometrium. She delivers a viable male infant weighing 3,560 gm with Apgar scores of 7 and 9 at one and five minutes of life, respectively.

The infant is admitted to the newborn nursery while G.K. recovers from anesthesia. G.K. is transferred to the postpartum care unit. She receives enoxaparin for deep vein thrombosis prophylaxis and 24 hours of intravenous magnesium sulfate for seizure prophylaxis.

G.K. has an uncomplicated postoperative course. Her blood pressures remain within normal limits. She and her infant son are discharged home on postoperative day three in stable condition.

Clinical Case Study 15.7

P.S. is a 34-year-old, G1 P0000 woman who is admitted to your labor and delivery unit at 34 weeks' gestation.

P.S. states that her amniotic membranes ruptured approximately two hours ago and the fluid was clear in color. She further states that she has been experiencing regular, painful uterine contractions since the membrane rupture. She denies decreased fetal movement.

You assist P.S. into bed and apply the electronic fetal monitor. You review with P.S. her prenatal record and note the following risk factors.

- History of chronic hypertension. She has been taking labetalol, 100 mg twice a day, for her blood pressure.
- History of infertility. This pregnancy was achieved by in-vitro fertilization with donor eggs.
- Allergy to sulfa drugs.

Your assessment of P.S. includes the following vital signs.

- Temperature: 37.1°C
- Pulse: 98 bpm
- Respirations: 20 rpm
- Blood pressure: 140/82 mmHg
- Pain rating: abdominal, 6/10

You notify P.S.'s care provider of her admission and your assessment. P.S.'s care provider performs a sterile speculum examination and obtains a vaginal/rectal culture for group B *Streptococcus* (GBS). The results from the sterile speculum examination include:

- positive pooling of clear amniotic fluid,
- positive nitrazine and fern test,
- cervix appears to be 2 cm dilated and approximately 50% effaced.

A bedside ultrasound confirms a vertex fetal presentation.

P.S. is diagnosed with preterm premature rupture of membranes (PPROM) with possible labor.

P.S. is tearful and states that she had hoped to have a normal pregnancy and delivery. She especially wants to breastfeed as soon as possible following delivery. Now she is afraid that she won't be able to do that. You provide support and suggest that a visit with a member from the neonatal intensive care unit (NICU) would help to address her concerns.

The decision is made to continue to monitor P.S.'s fetal heart rate (FHR) and uterine contraction activity and to start a course of penicillin for GBS prophylaxis.

You initiate intravenous access and begin the penicillin course. You notify the NICU of P.S.'s admission and of her concerns. A representative comes and speaks with P.S. and her husband regarding her baby's care following delivery. P.S. states that she feels her concerns were addressed.

It is now six hours later and P.S.'s uterine contraction activity has increased. P.S. states that she would like epidural analgesia. You notify her care provider who performs a vaginal examination. You note that P.S.'s cervix is now 7 cm dilated, 80% effaced, and the presenting fetal part is at 0 station.

The FHR tracing seen in Figure 15.7 is obtained using a cardiotachometer and tocodynamometer following completion of the epidural.

1.   In columns 01 through 15, you document P.S.'s uterine contraction activity as:

   A.   every two to three minutes, lasting 80 to 90 seconds, with intensity to be determined by palpation.
   B.   every two to four minutes, lasting 60 to 70 seconds with intensity of 60 to 75 mmHg, and a resting tone of 30 mmHg to 35 mmHg.
   C.   every three to five minutes, lasting 80 to 90 seconds, with intensity to be determined by palpation.

2.   In columns 01 through 15, you document P.S.'s FHR as:

   A.   FHR baseline of 140 bpm, minimal variability (amplitude range greater than undetectable to less than or equal to 5 bpm), accelerations and variable decelerations present.
   B.   FHR baseline of 120 bpm, moderate variability (amplitude range of 6 to 25 bpm), and variable decelerations present.
   C.   FHR baseline of 130 bpm, variability increased, and late decelerations present.

3.   Based on your assessment of P.S.'s FHR, your nursing interventions would include: (Choose all that apply)

   A.   changing P.S.'s position to relieve umbilical cord compression.
   B.   administering an intravenous fluid bolus of lactated Ringer's solution.
   C.   administering oxygen via nonrebreather facemask at 10 L/min.
   D.   notifying P.S.'s care provider.
   E.   making no changes in her nursing care.

4.   You would categorize this FHR tracing as a Category II because of the presence of:

   A.   minimal FHR variability.
   B.   recurrent variable FHR decelerations.
   C.   no FHR accelerations.
   D.   late FHR decelerations.

5.   Components of variable FHR decelerations that suggest fetal well-being include:

    A.   the FHR decelerations generally last no longer than 40 to 60 seconds on a recurrent basis.
    B.   the return of the FHR to baseline is abrupt.
    C.   the baseline FHR is not increasing.
    D.   the FHR variability is not decreasing.
    E.   all of the above.
    F.   A, B, and C only.

6.   When monitoring the preterm fetus:

    A.   the FHR baseline may be slightly higher than in a full-term fetus.
    B.   during labor, it may have less reserves.
    C.   variable FHR decelerations may be less frequent due to an increase in Wharton's jelly.
    D.   all of the above.
    E.   A and B only.

Figure 15.7

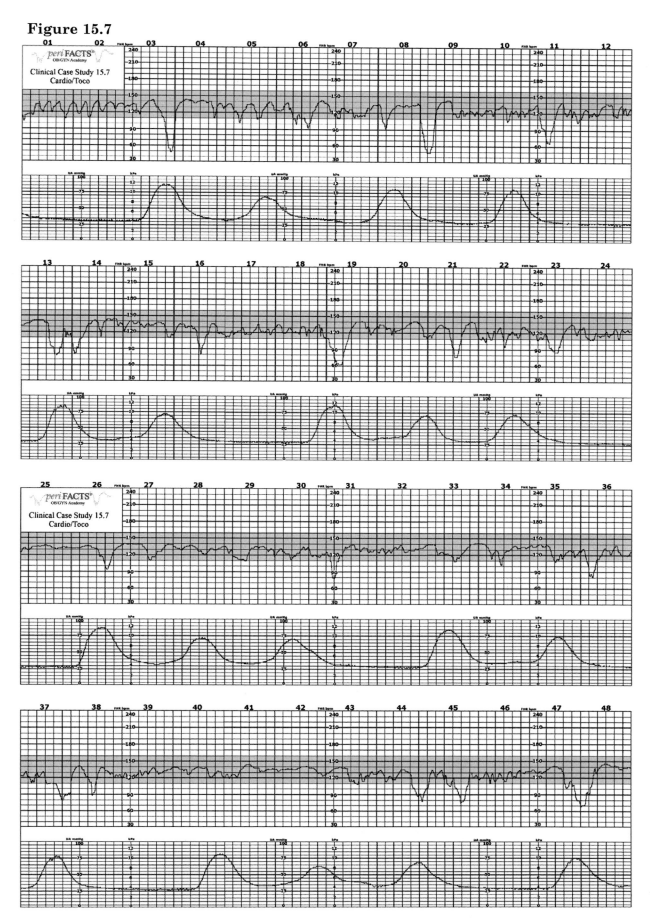

Clinical Case Study 15.7
Answers

1.   The correct answer is A.

2.   The correct answer is B.

3.   The correct answer is A, B, and D. At this point, oxygen administration is not indicated because of the presence of moderate variability, which indicates adequate oxygenation of the fetus.

4.   The correct answer is B.

5.   The correct answer is E.

6.   The correct answer is E.

OUTCOME

Within an hour of the end of this FHR tracing, P.S.'s cervix is fully dilated. After pushing for 15 minutes, P.S. spontaneously delivers a female infant weighing 1,815 gm with Apgar scores of 5 and 8 at one and five minutes, respectively. It is noted at delivery that there is a loose nuchal cord that is easily reduced. P.S.'s infant is handed to the neonatal intensive care unit (NICU) team. She is quickly assessed, and it is noted that her heart rate is less than 100 bpm. Positive pressure ventilation is initiated with room air, and her heart rate increases to greater than 100 bpm. P.S. and her husband are able to hold their baby for a few minutes before she is transferred to the NICU for prematurity and sepsis evaluation, which proves negative.

P.S.'s postpartum course is uncomplicated, and she is able to initiate breastfeeding on her first postpartum day. She is discharged home on her second postpartum day.

P.S.'s baby girl develops hyperbilirubinemia at 26 hours of life and requires phototherapy. By her fourth day of life, her hyperbilirubinemia has resolved and she is discharged home.

Glossary of Terms

periFACTS OB/GYN Academy's
Fetal Heart Rate Monitoring Glossary of Terms

Acceleration: An increase in fetal heart rate above baseline over less than 30 seconds. To be an acceleration, the peak must be greater than or equal to 15 bpm above the baseline, and must last greater than or equal to 15 seconds from the onset to return to baseline. Before 32 weeks' gestation, accelerations are defined as having a peak greater than or equal to 10 bpm above baseline and a duration of greater than or equal to 10 seconds.

Acidosis: Abnormal excess hydrogen ion concentration in tissues that is due to either increased acid buildup or increased loss of base.

> **Respiratory Acidosis:** A decrease in pH associated with an increase in carbonic acid and increase in PCO_2. HCO_3^- (bicarbonate) acutely rises but will normalize over time. The base deficit may be within normal range. If pulmonary or placental exchange is increased, the amount of CO_2 in the extracellular tissue may decrease.

> **Metabolic Acidosis:** Decrease in blood pH associated with an increase in hydrogen ions, decrease in PO_2 and HCO_3^-, and increase in base deficit (base excess). The PCO_2 usually is normal.

> **Mixed Acidosis:** Combination of metabolic and respiratory acidosis associated with a decrease in pH, decrease in PO_2, increase in PCO_2, and increase in base deficit.

Alkalosis: Abnormal decrease of hydrogen ion concentration in tissues that is due to either a decrease in acid or an accumulation of base.

Apgar Score: A system of scoring a neonate's physical condition after birth consisting of: heart rate, respiration, muscle tone, response to stimuli, and color, each receiving a 0, 1, or 2 for a maximum total score of 10.

Artifact: Inaccurate recording in the fetal heart rate.

Asphyxia (Fetal): Organ damage due to lack of oxygen.

Base Excess: The amount of base buffer reserves present either above or below normal levels. A large base deficit (e.g., -10 mEq/L) indicates that base buffers have been used to buffer acids and that metabolic acidosis is present.

Baseline Change: A change in the fetal heart rate that lasts greater than or equal to ten minutes, may result in a tachycardia or bradycardia.

Baseline Fetal Heart Rate: The mean fetal heart rate rounded to an increment of 5 bpm during a ten-minute window, excluding accelerations, decelerations, and marked variability. There must be at least two minutes of identifiable baseline segments (not necessarily continuous) in a ten-minute window or the baseline is indeterminate. Normally between 110 to 160 bpm.

Bradycardia: Baseline fetal heart rate less than 110 bpm for more than ten minutes.

Bishop's Score: A scoring system used to assess whether an induction of labor will produce a successful vaginal birth with a score of 9 suggesting a high likelihood of a successful induction.

Cervical Assessment

Cervical Effacement (also called cervical ripening): Refers to a thinning of the cervix. It is a component of the Bishop score. Prior to effacement, the cervix is like a long bottleneck, usually about four centimeters in length. Throughout pregnancy, the cervix is closed tightly and protected by a plug of mucus.

Cervical Dilation (or **cervical dilatation**): The opening of the cervix, the entrance to the uterus.

Contraction Stress Test (CST): A test used to assess the fetal-placental respiratory reserve by evaluating the fetal heart rate response to uterine contractions. The underlying premise is that a borderline-oxygenated fetus will demonstrate late decelerations when under stress induced by uterine contractions. It requires three contractions lasting 40 to 60 seconds in duration over a ten-minute period of observation of the fetal heart rate.

Equivocal: Decelerations that occur in the presence of uterine contractions more frequent than every two minutes or last longer than 90 seconds.

Equivocal—Suspicious: Intermittent late decelerations or significant variable decelerations.

Negative CST: No late or significant variable decelerations during a CST.

Positive CST: Late decelerations with 50% or more of contractions during a CST.

Unsatisfactory: Fewer than three contractions in a ten-minute period or an uninterpretable tracing.

Decelerations: A decrease in fetal heart rate below the baseline. These may be early, late, or variable in character.

Early Decelerations: Visually apparent, usually symmetric, gradual (onset to nadir greater than 30 seconds) decrease and return of the FHR associated with a uterine contraction. The nadir of the decelerations generally occurs coincident with the peak of the uterine contractions.

Intermittent Decelerations: Decelerations that occur with less than 50% of uterine contractions in any 20-minute window.

Late Decelerations: Visually apparent, usually symmetric, gradual (onset to nadir greater than 30 seconds) decrease and return of the FHR associated with a uterine contraction. The deceleration is delayed in timing, with the nadir of the deceleration occurring after the peak of the contraction.

Prolonged Deceleration: A decrease in fetal heart rate from the baseline greater than or equal to 15 bpm, lasting greater than or equal to two minutes, but less than ten minutes.

Recurrent Decelerations: Decelerations that occur with greater than or equal to 50% of uterine contractions in any 20-minute window.

Variable Decelerations: Visually apparent abrupt (onset to nadir less than 30 seconds) decrease in FHR. The decrease in fetal heart rate is greater than or equal to 15 bpm, lasting greater than or equal to 15 seconds, and less than two minutes in duration.

Episodic Changes: Accelerations and/or decelerations occurring without relationship to uterine contractions, such as during fetal movement.

Fetal Assessment

Fetal Presentation: Describes the part of the fetus that is descending into the pelvis.
- Cephalic: Vertex (head), sinciput (forehead), brow, face, or mentum (chin).
- Breech: Complete, footling, or frank (buttocks).
- Shoulder: Arm, shoulder, or trunk.

Fetal Attitude: The relationship of the fetal head to the fetal spine.
- Flexed (normal).
- Neutral (military).
- Extended.

Fetal Lie: The relationship of the longitudinal axis of the fetus to that of the mother.
- Longitudinal–Cephalic or breech.
- Oblique–Unstable lie–May go either longitudinal or transverse.
- Transverse–Shoulder.

Fetal Position: The relationship of the fetal presenting part to maternal pelvis. It is based on presentation.
- For example:
  - Vertex.
  - Left occiput anterior (LOA): Occiput is anterior and toward the left. Most common position.
  - Right occiput anterior (ROA): Occiput is anterior and toward the right.
  - Left occiput posterior (LOP): Occiput is posterior and toward the left.
  - Right occiput posterior (ROP): Occiput is posterior and toward the right.

Fetal Station: The degree of engagement from the presenting part to the ischial spines.
- Station 0: Presenting part is at the ischial spines.
- A negative number: The number of centimeters the presenting part is above the ischial spines.
- A positive number: The number of centimeters the presenting part is below the ischial spines.

Fetal Growth Restriction (FGR): Fetal growth below the 10th percentile for gestational age.

> **Asymmetric Fetal Growth Restriction:** Fetal growth restriction below the 10th percentile, that typically occurs later in pregnancy where the body proportions are altered to reflect redistribution of fetal blood flow to protect such vital organs as the brain. This often results in a normally grown head with a lagging abdominal circumference, and is also called "brain sparing" FGR.

> **Symmetric Fetal Growth Restriction:** FGR is growth restriction below the 10th percentile, usually beginning early in gestation where the fetal abdomen, head circumference, and femur-length measurements are all consistently small.

Fetal Heart Rate Interpretation System: A three-tier classification system for the interpretation of fetal heart rate (FHR) tracing developed by NICHD in 2008.

> **Category I Fetal Heart Rate Tracing:** Fetal heart rate tracings that include <u>all</u> of the following: (1) baseline rate: 110 to 160 bpm, (2) moderate baseline variability, (3) no late or variable decelerations, and (4) early decelerations and accelerations may or may not be present. Category I tracings are strongly predictive of normal fetal acid-base status at the time of observation.

> **Category II Fetal Heart Rate Tracing:** Fetal heart rate tracings that are indeterminate and are not predictive of abnormal fetal acid-base status, yet there is not adequate evidence at present to classify these as Category I or Category III.

> **Category III Fetal Heart Rate Tracing:** Fetal heart rate tracings that are either: (1) sinusoidal pattern, or (2) have absent baseline variability coupled with either recurrent late or variable decelerations or bradycardia. Category III tracings are predictive of abnormal fetal acid-base status at the time of observation.

Hypertonic Contractions: Contractions that plateau and do not return to baseline for two contraction cycles or five minutes, or one such contraction that lasts longer greater than or equal to two minutes.

Hypoxemia: Low levels of oxygen in blood.

Hypoxia: Low levels of oxygen in the tissue, inadequate to meet metabolic needs of the tissue.

Nonstress Test (NST): A fetal surveillance test based on the premise that a fetus with an intact, well-oxygenated central nervous system will accelerate its heart rate in response to fetal movement.

> **Reactive NST: 28 to 32 weeks' gestation:** NST that consists of <u>two</u> accelerations of the fetal heart rate 10 bpm above baseline, lasting ten seconds during a 20-minute period of observation.

> **Reactive NST: Greater than or equal to 32 weeks' gestation:** NST that consists of <u>two</u> accelerations of the fetal heart rate 15 bpm above baseline, lasting 15 seconds during a 20-minute period of observation.

> **Nonreactive NST:** NST that does not meet criteria for a reactive NST.

Periodic Changes: Accelerations and/or decelerations occurring in association with contractions.

Prolonged Acceleration: An acceleration lasting greater than or equal to two minutes but less than ten minutes in duration. An acceleration lasting longer than ten minutes is considered a baseline change.

Prolapsed Umbilical Cord: Expulsion of the umbilical cord into the vaginal canal ahead of the presenting fetal part.

Sinusoidal Fetal Heart Rate Pattern: A smooth, undulating pattern of uniform or fixed variability of the fetal heart rate that resembles a sine wave (~) and has a cycle frequency of 3 to 5 bpm that persists for greater than or equal to 20 minutes without areas of normal fetal heart rate variability or reactivity.

Tachycardia: Baseline fetal heart rate greater than 160 bpm for more than ten minutes.

Tachysystole: More than five uterine contractions within ten minutes, averaged over a 30-minute period.

Uterine Contraction Frequency (Normal): Less than or equal to five uterine contractions within ten minutes, averaged over a 30-minute period.

Uterine Resting Tone (Normal): The baseline tone of the uterus as measured by intrauterine pressure catheter, typically 8 to 12 mmHg.

Variability: The roughness or the smoothness of the line of the baseline fetal heart rate tracing.

> **Absent FHR Variability:** When the amplitude of the range in the baseline fetal heart rate is undetectable.

> **Minimal FHR Variability:** When the amplitude of the range in the baseline fetal heart rate is greater than undetectable but less than 5 bpm.

> **Moderate FHR Variability:** When the amplitude of the range in the baseline fetal heart rate is 6 to 25 bpm.

> **Marked FHR Variability:** When the amplitude of the range in the baseline fetal heart rate is greater than 25 bpm.

Appendices

1. Fetal Blood Gas Values
   - A.   Mean Umbilical Cord Blood Gas Values (Mean ± SD)
   - B.   Interpretation of Abnormal Fetal Blood Gas Values

2. Labor and Delivery
   - A.   Bishop's Score
   - B.   Positional Effects on Maternal Cardiac Output
   - C.   Hematologic Laboratory Assessment during Pregnancy
   - D.   Renal Laboratory Assessment during Pregnancy

3. Newborn Resuscitation
   - A.   Components of Apgar Scoring

4. Fetal Monitoring Interpretation
   - A.   NICHD: Definitions for Decelerations
   - B.   NICHD: Classification of Categories of Fetal Heart Rate Tracings
   - C.   Biophysical Profile Scoring Technique and Interpretation
   - D.   Interpretation of BPP Results and Recommended Clinical Management

1. Fetal Blood Gas Values

Appendix 1-A: Mean Umbilical Cord Blood Gas Values (Mean ± SD)

	Artery	Vein
pH	7.24 ± 0.07	7.32 ± 0.06
PCO_2 (mmHg)	56 ± 9	44 ± 7
PO_2 (mmHg)	18 ± 7	29 ± 7
BE (mEq/L)	-4 ± 3	-3 ± 2

Modified from Thorp (1989)

Appendix 1-B: Interpretation of Abnormal Fetal Blood Gas Values

Type of Acidosis	pH	PCO_2	HCO_3^-	Base Deficit
Respiratory	Decreased	Increased	Normal	Normal
Metabolic	Decreased	Normal	Decreased	Increased
Mixed	Decreased	Increased	Decreased	Increased

2. Labor and Delivery

Appendix 2-A: Bishop's Score

Cervix	0 points	1 point	2 points	3 points
Dilation (cm)	0	1 to 2	3 to 4	≥5
Effacement (%)	0 to 30	40 to 50	60 to 70	80 to 100
Station	-3	-2	-1, 0	+1, +2
Consistency	Firm	Medium	Soft	----------
Position	Posterior	Midposition	Anterior	----------

Appendix 2-B: Positional Effects on Maternal Cardiac Output

Position	Cardiac Output (L/min)
Knee chest	6.9
Right side	6.8
Left side	6.6
Sitting	6.2
Supine	6.0
Standing	5.4

Adapted from "Position change and central hemodynamic profile during normal third-trimester pregnancy and postpartum," American Journal of Obstetrics and Gynecology (1991).

Appendix 2-C: Hematologic Laboratory Assessment during Pregnancy
Note that these may vary by laboratory.

Test	Nonpregnant	Pregnant
Hematocrit	37% to 47%	33% to 44%
Hemoglobin	12 to 16 g/dL	11 to 14 g/dL
WBC count	4.5 to 11 x10^3/mm^3	6 to 16 x10^3/mm^3
Platelet count	130 to 400 x10^3/mm^3	Slight decrease
Fibrinogen	200 to 450 mg/dL	400 to 650 mg/dL
Prothrombin time (PT)	12 to 14 sec	Unchanged
Partial thromboplastin time (PTT)	24 to 36 sec	Unchanged

Appendix 2-D: Renal Laboratory Assessment during Pregnancy
Note that these may vary by laboratory

Test	Nonpregnant	Pregnant
Creatinine	<1.5 mg/dL	<0.8 mg/dL
BUN	10 to 20 mg/dL	5 to 12 mg/dL
Sodium	136 to 146 mEq/L	129 to 148 mEq/L
Potassium	3.5 to 5.0 mEq/L	3.3 to 5.0 mEq/L
CO_2 content	38 to 42 mEq/L	25 to 33 mEq/L
Calcium (total)	8.7 to 10.2 mg/dL	8.2 to 10.6 mg/dL
Glucose (fasting)	75 to 115 mg/dL	60 to 105 mg/dL
Uric acid	2.5 to 5.6 mg/dL	2.0 to 6.3 mg/dL

Adapted from Burrow and Duffy, 1999.

3. Newborn Resuscitation

Appendix 3-A: Components of Apgar Scoring

	Score of 0	Score of 1	Score of 2	Component of Acronym
Appearance/ Complexion	Blue or pale all over	Blue at extremities body pink (acrocyanosis)	No cyanosis body and extremities pink	Appearance
Pulse Rate	Absent	Less than 100 beats per minute	Greater than 100 beats per minute	Pulse
Reflex Irritability Grimace	No response to stimulation	Grimace on suction or aggressive stimulation	Cry on stimulation	Grimace
Activity	None	Some flexion	Flexed arms and legs that resist extension	Activity
Respiratory Effort	Absent	Weak, irregular, gasping	Strong, lusty cry	Respiratory

Apgar, Virginia (1953). A proposal for a new method of evaluation of the newborn infant. *Current researches in anesthesia & analgesia* 32(4):260–267.

4. Fetal Monitoring Interpretation

Appendix 4-A: NICHD: Definitions for Decelerations

Early Deceleration:
- Visually apparent, usually symmetric, *gradual* decrease and return of the fetal heart rate (FHR) associated with a uterine contraction.
- A *gradual* decrease in onset to nadir of greater than or equal to 30 seconds.
- The decrease is calculated from the onset to the nadir of the deceleration.
- The nadir of the deceleration occurs at the same time as the peak of the contraction.
- In most cases, the onset, nadir, and recovery of the deceleration are coincident with the beginning, peak, and ending of the contraction, respectively.

Variable Deceleration:
- Visually apparent *abrupt* decrease in FHR, defined as less than 30 seconds from the onset of the deceleration to the beginning of the nadir.
- The decrease in FHR is calculated from the onset to the nadir of the deceleration.
- The decrease in FHR is greater than or equal to 15 beats per minute, lasting greater than or equal to 15 seconds, but less than or equal to two minutes in duration.
- When associated with uterine contractions, their onset, depth, and duration commonly vary with successive uterine contractions.

Late Deceleration:
- Visually apparent usually symmetric gradual decrease and return of the fetal heart rate associated with a uterine contraction.
- A gradual FHR decrease is defined as from the onset to the FHR nadir of greater than or equal to 30 seconds.
- The decrease in FHR is calculated from the onset to the nadir of the deceleration.
- The deceleration is delayed in timing, with the nadir of the deceleration occurring after the peak of the contraction.

Adapted from: Macones GA, Hankins GDV, Spong CY, Hauth J, Moore T (2008). The 2008 National Institute of Child Health and Human Development Workshop Report on Electronic Fetal Monitoring: Update on Definitions, Interpretation, and Research Guidelines. American College of Obstetricians and Gynecologists, 112:661-6.

Appendix 4-B: NICHD: Classification of Categories of Fetal Heart Rate Tracings[∇]

Category I*

- Baseline rate between 110 to 160 beats per minutes (bpm)

- Moderate baseline variability

- Absent late or variable decelerations

- Presence or absence of early decelerations

- Presence or absence of accelerations

Category II[†]

- Bradycardia without absent baseline variability.
- Tachycardia
- Minimal baseline variability
- Absent baseline variability but without recurrent decelerations
- Marked baseline variability
- Absence of accelerations following fetal stimulation
- Recurrent variable decelerations with minimal or moderate baseline variability
- Prolonged deceleration lasting greater than or equal to two minutes but less than ten minutes
- Recurrent late decelerations with moderate baseline variability
- Variable decelerations associated with other characteristics such as slow return to baseline, "shoulders," or "overshoots"

Category III*

- Absent baseline variability associated with:
  - Recurrent late decelerations
  - Recurrent variable decelerations
  - Bradycardia
- Sinusoidal pattern

*These tracings include all of the following patterns.

[†]These tracings include, but are not limited to, the following patterns. Additionally, this category includes patterns not classified as Category I or III.

∇ Adapted from: Macones GA, Hankins GDV, Spong CY, Hauth J, Moore T (2008). The 2008 National Institute of Child Health and Human Development Workshop Report on Electronic Fetal Monitoring: Update on Definitions, Interpretation, and Research Guidelines. American College of Obstetricians and Gynecologists, 112:661-6.

Appendix 4-C: Biophysical Profile Scoring Technique and Interpretation

Biophysical Variable	Normal (score=2)	Abnormal (score =0)
Fetal breathing movements	Greater than or equal to one episode of greater than or equal to 30 sec in 30 min.	Absent or no episode of greater than or equal to 30 sec in 30 min.
Gross body movements	Greater than or equal to three discrete body/limb movements in 30 min (episodes of active continuous movement considered one movement).	Less than three episodes of body/limb movements in 30 min as single movement.
Fetal tone	Greater than or equal to one episode of active extension with return to flexion of fetal limb(s) or trunk. Opening and closing of hand considered normal tone.	Either slow extension with return to partial flexion, movement of limb in full extension, or absent fetal movement.
Reactive fetal heart rate	Two accelerations in 20-minute period. For fetuses greater than or equal to 32 weeks' gestation, greater than or equal to 15 bpm and of greater than or equal to 15 seconds duration. For fetuses less than 32 weeks' gestation, greater than or equal to 10 bpm and of greater than or equal to ten seconds duration.	Insufficient accelerations, absent accelerations in a 20-minute tracing.
Qualitative amniotic fluid volume	Greater than or equal to one pocket of fluid measuring 2x2 cm in vertical axis.	Either no pockets or largest pocket less than 2 cm in vertical axis.

Appendix 4-D: Interpretation of BPP Results and Recommended Clinical Management

Test Score Result	Risk Asphyxia	Perinatal Morbidity Within One Week Without Intervention	Management	% Fetal Acidemia	Corrected Mortality per 1,000
10 of 10, 8 of 10 (normal fluid), 8 of 8 (NST not done)	Risk of fetal asphyxia extremely rare	1 per 1,000	Intervention only for obstetric and maternal factors, not fetal.	13	1
8 of 10 (low fluid)	Possible chronic fetal compromise	89 per 1,000	If fetal kidneys present and intact membranes; deliver for fetal indications; if preterm, consider continued surveillance	No data	No data
6 of 10 (normal fluid)	Equivocal test, possible fetal asphyxia	Variable	Deliver if mature, in the immature fetus, repeat within 24 hr; if persistent, deliver	24	10
6 out of 10 (low fluid)	Probable fetal asphyxia	89 per 1,000	Deliver for fetal indications	No data	No data
4 of 10	High probability for fetal asphyxia	91 per 1,000	Consider CST if immature; deliver if mature	58	26
2 of 10	Fetal asphyxia almost certain	125 per 1,000	Deliver if greater than or equal to 32 weeks	67	94
0 of 10	Fetal asphyxia certain	600 per 1,000	Deliver if greater than or equal to 32 weeks	100	285

Adapted from:
Manning FA, Platt LD, and Sipos L (1980). Antepartum fetal evaluation: development of a fetal biophysical profile score. American Journal of Obstetrics and Gynecology, 136:787.
Manning FA. Chapter 23 Fetal Biophysical Profile Score: Theoretical Considerations and Practical Application IN: Sonography in Obstetrics and Gynecology: Seventh Edition. Fleischer, Toy, Lee, Manning, Romero Ed. McGraw-Hill Professional; 2011.

Index

Index